Lactate Threshold Training

Peter Janssen, MD

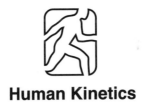

Human Kinetics

Library of Congress Cataloging-in-Publication Data

Janssen, Peter G. J. M., 1942-
   Lactate threshold training/by Peter G.J.M. Janssen.
     p. cm.
   Includes bibliographical references and index.
   ISBN 0-7360-3755-1
     1. Sports--Physiological aspects. 2. Physical education and training. I. Title.

   RC1235 .J36 2001
   612'.044--dc21   00-054237

ISBN: 0-7360-3755-1

This book is a revised edition of *Hetnieuwe BasisBoek Training*, published in 1999 by Kosmos-Z & K Uitgevers, Utrecht/Antwerpen.

Acquisitions Editor: Martin Barnard; **Developmental Editor:** Patricia Norris, PhD; **Managing Editor:** Wendy McLaughlin; **Assistant Editor:** Dan Brachtesende; **Copyeditor:** Julie Anderson; **Proofreader:** Myla Smith; **Indexer:** Marie Rizzo; **Permission Manager:** Toni Harte; **Graphic Designer:** Nancy Rasmus; **Graphic Artist:** Dody Bullerman; **Photo Manager:** Clark Brooks; **Cover Designer:** Jack Davis; **Photographer (cover):** © David Madison/Bruce Coleman, Inc.; **Photographer (interior):** Tom Roberts, unless otherwise noted; **Art Manager:** Craig Newsom; **Illustrator:** Mic Greenberg; **Printer:** United Graphics

Human Kinetics books are available at special discounts for bulk purchase. Special editions or book excerpts can also be created to specification. For details, contact the Special Sales Manager at Human Kinetics.

Printed in the United States of America   10 9 8 7 6 5 4 3 2 1

Human Kinetics
Web site: **www.humankinetics.com**

United States: Human Kinetics
P.O. Box 5076
Champaign, IL 61825-5076
800-747-4457
e-mail: humank@hkusa.com

Canada: Human Kinetics
475 Devonshire Road Unit 100
Windsor, ON N8Y 2L5
800-465-7301 (in Canada only)
e-mail: orders@hkcanada.com

Europe: Human Kinetics, P.O. Box IW14
Leeds LS16 6TR, United Kingdom
+44 (0) 113 278 1708
e-mail: humank@hkeurope.com

Australia: Human Kinetics
57A Price Avenue
Lower Mitcham, South Australia 5062
08 8277 1555
e-mail: liahka@senet.com.au

New Zealand: Human Kinetics
P.O. Box 105-231, Auckland Central
09-523-3462
e-mail: hkp@ihug.co.nz

Lactate Threshold Training

contents

	Preface	vi
	Key	vii
Chapter 1	**Energy**	**1**
	Energy systems	
	Energy stores	
	Types of muscle fibers	
	Targeted training	
Chapter 2	**Heart Rate**	**25**
	Counting the heart rate	
	Maximum heart rate	
	Conconi's method	
	Factors influencing heart rate	
Chapter 3	**The Deflection Point**	**65**
	Conconi's test	
	Åstrand test	
	Maximal test	
	Finding the deflection point	
	Individual anaerobic threshold test	
Chapter 4	**Lactate**	**107**
	The lactate curve	
	Blood lactate measurement	
	Practical applications of the lactate test	
Chapter 5	**Overtraining**	**151**
	Supercompensation	
	The lactate paradox	
	Causes of overtraining	
	Some specific health problems	

Chapter 6	**Circulation**	**165**
	The heart	
	The heart minute volume	
	Stroke volume	
	The sports heart	

Chapter 7	**Blood Levels**	**175**
	Characteristics of blood	
	Decrease in oxygen transport	
	Optimizing oxygen transport	
	Hematocrit	

Chapter 8	**Nutrition**	**205**
	Energy	
	Sources of energy	
	Nutrition for endurance sports	
	Energy consumption for events	
	Fluid and endurance sports	

Chapter 9	**Heart Rate Patterns**	**229**
	Lactate determination	
	Comparisons of performance capacity	
	Heart rate patterns of various workouts	

Epilogue	285
Glossary	288
Bibliography	291
Index	297
About the Author	303

preface

The impetus for this book was the spectacular improvement of the world hour record in cycling by the Italian Francesco Moser. In 1984, he smashed the previously unassailable record of Eddy Merckx and was the first to break the magic limit of 50 kilometers. Since that time the record has been broken again: On September 6, 1996, Chris Boardman rode 56.375 kilometers in Manchester, England. The explanation for these enormous achievements, which had been deemed impossible for a long time, can be found in the training principles of the physiology professor Francesco Conconi, who then coached Francesco Moser. Conconi developed a special training method centered on heart rate at the same time the heart rate monitor was developed in Finland. From that point onward, every athlete could improve his or her achievements with the help of specific training guidelines.

Moser's success and the later successes of Italian cyclists and endurance athletes have contributed to the worldwide acceptance of Conconi's training principles. Heart rate monitoring of workouts and races, with or without lactate determination, is now essential to athletes and coaches. Conconi's method is applicable to both elite and recreational athletes. This book was written for athletes, but also for trainers, sports physicians, and other coaches who need to know how to improve performance. The Conconi principle is simple yet so universal to endurance sports that every endurance athlete and coach should become familiar with it.

The book covers both theory and practice. The principles of energy supply are explained and applied to practical programs. All relevant tests are described, from laboratory tests to simple self-tests. Forms of training and training advice are explained in detail, and races and workouts are analyzed and evaluated. Essential advice on nutrition, overtraining, and the training the athlete's heart is also included.

bpm	beats per min
HR	heart rate
L	lactate
mmol	millimoles
W	watt
g	gram
l	liter
m	meter
km	kilometer
sec	second
min	minute
h	hour
d	day
mo	month
V	velocity

Conversions

1 mile = 1.61 kilometers/ 0.62 kilometers = 1 mile

1 kilocalorie = 4.184 kilojoules

1 pound = 16 ounces/ .454 kilograms = 1 pound

1 ounce = 28.35 grams

0 C = 32° F

chapter 1

Energy

Muscles at work need energy. Thus, any exercise requires an energy supply. There are different energy-supplying systems, and each system has its own characteristics. Drawing up an optimal training program is possible only when the principles of energy supply are well understood.

It is possible to feel within one's own body which system is stressed to supply the working muscles with energy. In everyday practice, however, many athletes do not follow their bodies' cues so that they can adjust their programs accordingly. Many athletes train too intensively or with too little variation, whereas others work with too little intensity, and so they never reach the desired effects. The optimal training intensity can be established with the help of lactate determinations and heart rate (HR) recordings; this often enables athletes to improve, with even less training.

Energy Systems

Three systems supply energy to working muscles. Muscles are driven by phosphates, oxygen, and lactate. The intensity of exercise determines which energy system is used.

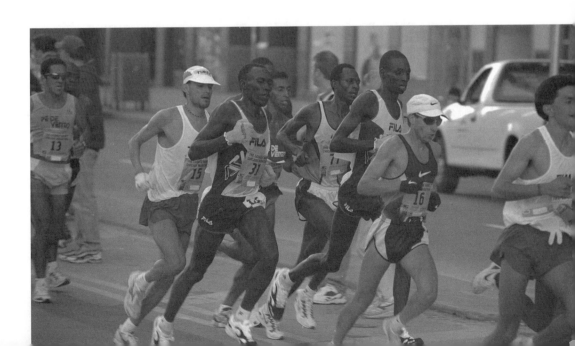

The Phosphate System

The phosphate system supplies energy directly; it does not need oxygen and does not produce lactic acid. Within the body there is a high-energy chemical substance called adenosine triphosphate (ATP) that enables muscles to contract. During muscular activity this compound is broken down to adenosine diphosphate (ADP), which supplies the muscle with direct energy.

$$ATP \rightarrow ADP + energy$$

The ATP store in the muscles is limited, but fortunately a number of aiding systems within the muscle are constantly busy resynthesizing ATP from the ADP produced. This process of resynthesis maintains a constant amount of ATP so that the muscle can keep working.

An important aiding system is creatine phosphate (CP). The store of this substance is limited, but it is capable of resynthesizing ATP from ADP very quickly.

$$CP + ADP \rightarrow ATP + creatine$$

Because of the limited store of CP, this aiding system cannot offer a lasting solution. The amount of ATP in store is sufficient for about 2 seconds of maximum effort, and the amount of CP is greatly reduced after some 6 to 8 seconds. Energy supply via this route is then ineffective.

As mentioned, the phosphate system needs no oxygen and produces no lactic acid. The energy supplied by this system is directly available. At a maximum effort this system is exhausted within 10 seconds, and it supplies energy for only 6 to 8 seconds. The supply of energy is possible through ATP present in the muscle and through the breakdown of CP, and it takes place at the onset of any activity. This system is important for the starts of sprinters, football players, jumpers, discus throwers, boxers, and tennis players—that is, explosive, short, rapid, and powerful activities.

The resynthesis of CP after the activity ends is also very fast. The store of high-energy phosphates (ATP + CP) that was exhausted during physical activity is replenished within a few minutes after the activity is finished. This process is 70% complete within 30 seconds and 100% after 3 to 5 minutes.

The phosphate system is trained by fierce, short power explosions, alternated with periods of rest. These periods of rest should be long enough for ATP and CP to resynthesize (see graph 1).

ATP and CP stores increase by 25% to 50% after 7 months of endurance training that consists of running three times a week. ATP and CP are the most rapidly accessible sources of energy. An increase in ATP and CP increases the athlete's capacity to succeed in activities that last only about 10 seconds.

Eight weeks of sprint training increases the enzymes that break down and rebuild ATP. Thus, ATP is broken down much faster and energy is released more quickly. So training not only increases ATP and CP stores but also speeds the process of breaking down and rebuilding ATP. These adaptations—the

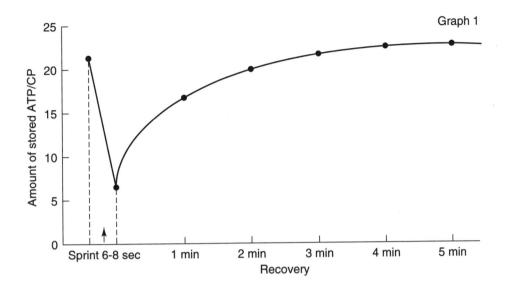

Graph 1

increase of ATP and CP and the enhanced enzyme activity—are brought about by well-chosen endurance and sprint training programs.

The Oxygen System

The oxygen system, also called the aerobic system, is an aiding system that burns nutrients. A lasting, non-time-related form of energy supply, resynthesis of ATP, is offered by the reaction of mainly carbohydrates and fats with oxygen. These nutrients are taken in with normal food consumption and are stored in depots to be used when needed. In terms of energy, the store of fats is practically unlimited. Carbohydrates—sugars, starches, and glucose—are stored in the liver and the muscles in the form of glycogen. The store of glycogen may vary widely, but in most cases it is sufficient for at least 60 to 90 minutes of submaximal exercise. The breakdown of fats is as follows:

Fats + oxygen + ADP → carbon dioxide + ATP + water

Carbon dioxide is removed by the lungs. The breakdown of carbohydrates, called glycolysis, is somewhat more complex. It takes place in two successive reactions, shown as follows:

First phase: glucose + ADP → lactic acid + ATP

Second phase: lactic acid + oxygen + ADP → carbon dioxide + ATP + water

The first phase does not use oxygen, whereas the second does. When the exercise is light, the by-product lactic acid (also called lactate) is directly worked in the second phase, so that the final result is as follows:

Glucose + oxygen + ADP → carbon dioxide + ATP + water

If, during exercise, the oxygen system is not stressed beyond certain limits, the inhaled oxygen is sufficient and lactic acid does not accumulate. At the beginning of exercise, the body uses the aerobic energy supply—carbohydrates, fats, and proteins. It takes 2 to 3 minutes before the heart, lungs, and blood circulation fully function (see graph 2).

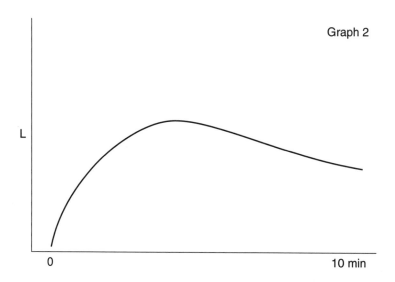

Graph 2

The store of carbohydrates is limited, whereas the store of fats is practically unlimited. The two systems work simultaneously, but their contributions to energy supply are different and, moreover, depend greatly on the level of exertion and training.

Fats are burned during low-intensity exercise. As intensity increases, carbohydrate oxidation becomes more important as a source of energy. After a period of training, energy is used more economically. This means that the well-trained athlete burns fats for a longer time, thus saving carbohydrates. Training may increase aerobic capacity by 50% (see graph 3).

The Lactate System

As the level of exertion increases, the body reaches a point at which the oxygen system cannot keep up anymore. This is when the anaerobic or lactate system begins to produce lactic acid. At this point, the demand for energy overstresses the second phase of the oxygen system. The second phase of the oxygen system is unable to neutralize the lactic acid formed in the first phase, and the accumulation of lactic acid increases in the working muscles, which is a condition known as acidosis.

$$Glucose + ADP \rightarrow lactic\ acid + ATP$$

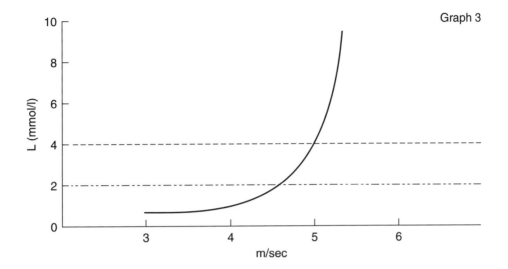

Graph 3

Muscle soreness is characteristic of increasing acidosis (e.g., sore legs for the cyclist or runner or sore arms for the rower). With increasing acidosis, the athlete cannot maintain the same level of exercise. Whenever the cyclist or runner must let the pack go, acidosis is most likely the cause. The athlete who can delay the moment of acidosis longest will probably win the race.

When a certain level of intensity (which differs from one person to another) is surpassed, a kind of emergency system becomes active whereby the body draws on the anaerobic energy supply, which uses only carbohydrates as a fuel. Within seconds or minutes, depending on the athlete's level of training, exercise intensity decreases drastically or activity even stops because of the accumulation of lactate, which results in increasing muscle fatigue.

For exertions of short duration, such as the 100-, 200-, 400-, and 800-meter runs and other very intensive activities that last 2 to 3 minutes, the energy supply used is mainly anaerobic. In the 1,500-meter run, energy supply is about 50% aerobic and about 50% anaerobic. At the onset of any exercise, independent of its intensity, energy supply is always anaerobic and lactic. It always takes some minutes before the aerobic system functions completely— before respiration, heart rate, and the transport of oxygen through the blood adjust to the demands of the activity. Until that time, at the beginning of the exercise, the lactate system supplies the necessary energy.

The lactate system also supplies the energy during increases of pace that surpass the aerobic level in an otherwise normal endurance exertion, such as surges, climbing, and escapes. Also, in the final sprint after an exertion of long duration (for example, at the finish of a marathon or a cycling race), the lactate system supplies the extra energy (see graph 4).

The high lactate values that may arise during heavy exercise can be disadvantageous. These high lactate values are proof that the aerobic energy

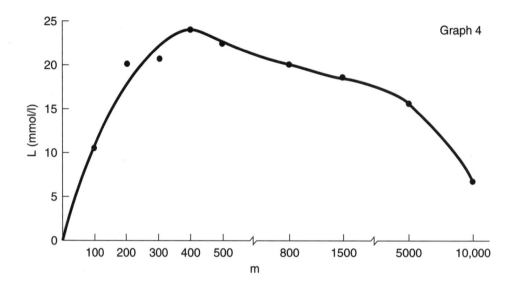

supply is failing. The anaerobic energy supply, which meets the deficiency, has lactic acid as a by-product. The maximum lactate content that can be reached might well be 20 times the value at rest.

High lactate values cause muscle fatigue. When an athlete begins an endurance run at a pace that is too high or begins the final sprint too soon, lactic acid content will increase to high values. The fatigue that follows increased lactic acid will cause the athlete to lose the race.

High lactate values cause acidosis in and around the muscle cells. This acidosis may seriously disturb various mechanisms within the muscle cells. The system of aerobic enzymes in the muscle cell may be seen as a factory where aerobic energy supply is generated. This enzyme system is damaged by acidosis, which decreases aerobic endurance capacity. After acidosis damage, it may take days before this system recovers sufficiently and regains aerobic capacity. When the exercise is repeatedly too intensive (i.e., without sufficient recovery), aerobic endurance capacity decreases considerably. These overly-intensive workouts then lead to a complex of complaints called overtraining. Acidosis damages the wall of the muscle cell, causing a leakage from the muscle cell into the blood. The day after a heavy workout all kinds of abnormalities can be seen in the blood, especially higher values of ureum, creatine kinase, aspartate aminotransferase, and alanine aminotransferase, which all indicate damage of the muscle cell wall.

It may take 24 to 96 hours before these values are normalized again, and should be taken into consideration when choosing the type of workout. In this situation, training should be light: the so-called recovery or regeneration workout. If training is too intensive, recovery will take much longer.

High lactate values disturb coordination capacity. Intensive training in combination with high lactate values disturbs the contraction mechanism within the muscle and therefore also affects coordination capacity, which is important in sports that require much technical skill (e.g., tennis, football, and judo). Technique training should never be performed with lactate values more than 6 to 8 millimoles per liter, because coordination is then so disturbed that technique training will not be effective.

High lactate values enhance injury risk. The acidosis within the muscle causes microruptures (minor damages that can lead to injuries if recovery is insufficient.) In the presence of high lactate values, the formation of CP is delayed, which is a reason to avoid high lactate values during sprint workouts.

At high lactate values, the burning of fats decreases. When glycogen reserves are depleted, energy supply is endangered at high lactate values because fat cannot be used as an energy source.

When the body is at rest, it takes about 25 minutes to remove half the accumulated lactate that results from maximal exertion; 95% of the lactate is removed after 1 hour and 15 minutes. After heavy to maximal exercise, lactate is removed from blood and muscles

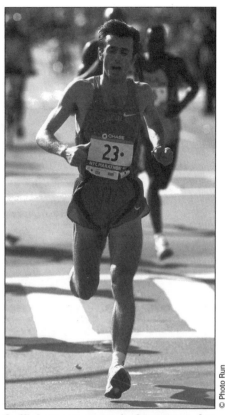

Sufficient recovery is important for marathoners like Giacome Leone.

much more quickly when light work is done during the recovery phase instead of complete rest. This so-called active recovery is, in fact, no more than the cool-down activity that most athletes perform. As shown in graph 5, an

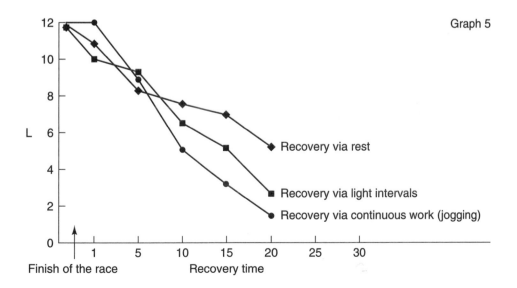

Graph 5

Recovery via rest

Recovery via light intervals

Recovery via continuous work (jogging)

L

Finish of the race   Recovery time

active recovery such as jogging decreases lactate most quickly. The graph also shows that during this recovery phase, it is best to do continuous work instead of intervals.

Tables 1.1 through 1.4 summarize the activities of the three energy systems.

Table 1.1 Substrates for Energy Supply and Their Characteristics

Substrate production	Process	Availability	Speed of energy
CP	Anaerobic alactic	Very limited	Very fast
Glycogen or glucose	Anaerobic lactic	Limited	Fast
Fatty acids	Aerobic alactic	Unlimited	Very slow

Energy supply	Anaerobic alactic	Anaerobic lactic	Aerobic alactic
Energy via	ATP/CP	Glycolysis	Reaction with oxygen
Supplies	Direct energy	2-3 mmol ATP	36 mmol ATP
Time	6-8 sec	6-8 sec to 2-3 min	Longer than 2-3 min
By product	No lactate formed	Lactate	No lactate formed
Name	Phosphate system	Lactate system	Oxygen system
Activity	Onset of exercise	Short and fierce surges	Long-lasting exercise
Sprint examples	Short sprints	Closing a gap 1-km time trial 400- to 800-m run	Long time trial marathon Long distances
Capacity	Sprint capacity	Tolerance	Endurance

Table 1.2 Qualities of the Three Systems of ATP Synthesis

System	Food or chemical fuel	Oxygen needed	Speed	ATP production
Anaerobic ATP/CP system	Creatine phosphate	No	Fastest	Little, limited
Lactic acid system	Glycogen (glucose)	No	Fast	Little, limited
Aerobic oxygen system	Glycogen, fats, proteins	Yes	Slow	Much, limited

Table 1.3 Maximum Workload of Various Durations in Relation to Energy Supply

Duration	Classification	Energy source	Remarks
1-5 sec	Anaerobic alactic	ATP	
6-8 sec	Anaerobic alactic	ATP + CP	
9-45 sec	Anaerobic alactic + anaerobic lactic	ATP, CP + muscle glycogen	High lactate production
45-120 sec	Anaerobic lactic	Muscle glycogen	As duration increases, lactate production decreases
120-240 sec	Aerobic + anaerobic lactic	Muscle glycogen	
240-600 sec	Aerobic	Muscle glycogen + fatty acids	Higher share of fatty acids, increasing duration

Table 1.4 Maximum Amount and Maximum Capacity of the Three Energy Systems

System	Maximum capacity* (mol ATP/min)	Maximum amount** (total amount ATP in mol)
ATP/CP (phosphate system)	3.6	0.7
Anaerobic glycolysis (lactate system)	1.6	1.2
Aerobic or oxygen system (only on glycogen)	1.0	90.0

*The amount in one time unit.
**The amount independent of time.

Summary of various forms of energy supply

a. ATP = ADP + energy anaerobic, alactic

b. CP + ADP = creatine + ATP anaerobic, alactic

c. glucose + ADP = lactic acid + ATP anaerobic, lactic

d. glucose + oxygen + ADP = water, carbon dioxide + ATP aerobic, alactic

e. fat + oxygen + ADP = water, carbon dioxide + ATP aerobic, alactic

Aerobic: using oxygen

Anaerobic: without using oxygen

Lactic: producing lactic acid

Alactic: without producing lactic acid

ATP-CP → phosphate system = a + b

Anaerobic glycolysis → lactate system = c

Aerobic glycolysis → oxygen system = d + e

Energy Stores

The store of ATP is exhausted after 4 seconds of maximum effort. CP is totally consumed after 8 to 10 seconds of maximum effort, and the glycogen store is depleted after 60 to 90 minutes of submaximal effort. The amount of fat available for energy supply is unlimited (see graph 6).

Fats supply 9 kilocalories per gram and carbohydrates supply 4 kilocalories. Stored fats are not combined with water, although stored carbohydrates are combined with a considerable amount of water. If the energy stored within our bodies in the form of fats should be replaced by carbohydrates, our body weights would double. That is the reason why birds of passage only store fats as a fuel. So, per weight unit, fat is an efficient source of energy. It is the ideal fuel for long-duration efforts when food intake is limited.

The total carbohydrate store is between 8,000 and 12,000 kilojoules (2,000 and 3,000 kilocalories). The human body has an enormous capacity to store fats, although the store of fats may vary widely. A man has a mean fat percentage between 10% and 20%; for a woman, this is between 20% and 30%.

Well-trained endurance athletes have a mean fat percentage of about 10%. The ideal fat percentage may differ from athlete to athlete, ranging from extremely low percentages (4% to 5%) to somewhat higher values (12% to

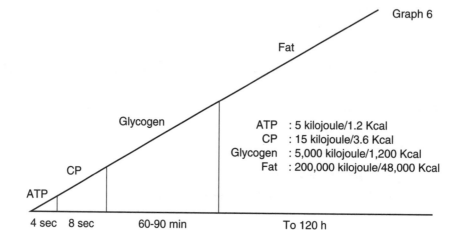

Graph 6

Fat

Glycogen

CP

ATP

ATP	: 5 kilojoule/1.2 Kcal
CP	: 15 kilojoule/3.6 Kcal
Glycogen	: 5,000 kilojoule/1,200 Kcal
Fat	: 200,000 kilojoule/48,000 Kcal

4 sec   8 sec   60-90 min   To 120 h

13%). But every athlete has his or her own ideal fat percentage, which does not change, and this fat percentage is an important parameter of the athlete's condition. A too high or too low fat percentage will prevent the athlete from reaching top condition.

The average carbohydrate store supplies energy for 95 minutes of marathon running, whereas the store of fats is depleted after 119 hours. But the burning of fats consumes more oxygen. Per time unit, more ATP can be formed out of carbohydrates than out of fats. Therefore, carbohydrates are the most important source of energy during intensive exercise. When the carbohydrate store becomes exhausted, the burning of fats increases and the level of intensity decreases. In the marathon this often happens around the 30-kilometer mark, after some 90 minutes of running.

Types of Muscle Fibers

Every muscle consists of different types of muscle fibers. The fibers are very different in function, but they all must be supplied with energy. It is important to understand the differences in the fibers, because every muscle fiber requires specific training.

The red, or slow, fibers are also called Type I or slow-twitch fibers. The white, or fast, fibers are also called Type II or fast-twitch fibers. There are no differences between men and women in the relation between the fast-twitch and slow-twitch fibers. Trainability for women is the same as for men.

The Red Muscle Fibers

The richly capillaried red muscle fibers have a mainly aerobic energy supply. Therefore, the red fibers have a great aerobic capacity and a limited anaerobic capacity, making them important for stamina. They work rather slowly and do not fatigue easily, so they are able to keep working for a long time during endurance exercise.

The White Muscle Fibers

The moderately capillaried white muscle fibers have a mainly anaerobic energy supply. The white fibers have a great anaerobic capacity and a rather small aerobic capacity, so the white fiber system is important for explosiveness or sprinting capacity. The white fibers work fast and therefore are easily exhausted. Fierce efforts that call on the white fibers can only be maintained for a short period of time.

The white fibers, the type II fibers, can be subdivided into Type IIa and Type IIb fibers. The Type IIa fibers can supply aerobic energy in addition to their anaerobic function, and in so doing they support the type I fibers during endurance exercise. The Type IIb fibers are clearly anaerobic and have hardly any function during an endurance workout.

The Red/White Muscle Fiber Ratio

The higher the number of fast-twitch fibers, the better the athlete's sprinting capacity. The slow-twitch and fast-twitch fiber ratio may vary widely among people, but the muscle fiber ratio in any person is basically unchangeable. So you are born to be a sprinter or an endurance athlete. In a sprinter, the slow-twitch/fast-twitch fiber ratio is 50/50, whereas a marathon runner may have a slow-twitch/fast-twitch ratio of 90/10. Graph 7 shows typical ratios for different types of athletes.

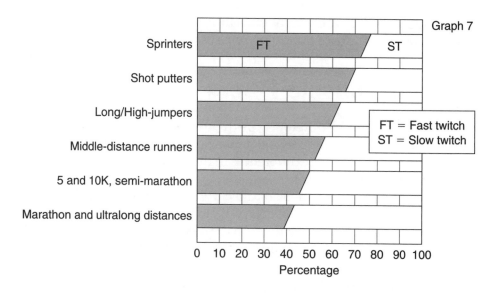

Muscle fiber composition determines whether somebody is an explosive or endurance type of athlete. But the system is not totally immutable. By following a well-targeted training program, explosive athletes such as sprinters can develop their endurance capacity. The correct training can increase the number of red fibers, which then alters the ratio of red and white fibers. Simply said, the training stimulus can rebuild white fibers into red fibers.

The opposite is impossible. An endurance athlete cannot change his or her muscle fiber pattern by performing sprinting workouts. Pronounced endurance athletes will always be weak sprinters. Sprinters, however, might very well develop into good endurance athletes, although their improvement in endurance will decrease the power of their sprint.

As athletes age, sprinting capacity decreases faster than endurance capacity. It is most likely that sprinting performance will decrease with a decrease in the number of fast-twitch fibers. Endurance capacity can be maintained until advanced age.

Fiber Type and Exercise Intensity

Light exercise, such as walking, easy cycling, or jogging, can be maintained for many hours. Energy supply is then fully aerobic, through fat oxidation in the Type I fibers. The store of fats is practically inexhaustible.

With intermediate exercise, such as running or cycling, all Type I fibers may soon become active. Beside fat oxidation, there is an increasing share of carbohydrate oxidation, although energy supply is still completely aerobic. Well-trained athletes can maintain maximum aerobic effort for 1 to 2 hours, after which the store of carbohydrates is exhausted.

With a further increase in intensity, as in a time trial or a 10-kilometer run, the Type IIa fibers begin to support aerobic energy supply, and carbohydrates are oxidized maximally. The complete aerobic system is actively supplying energy, but the anaerobic system also supplies its share of energy. This anaerobic energy supply has lactic acid as a by-product. Up to a certain level of intensity, there is an equilibrium between the formation and the breakdown of lactic acid. The body is capable of breaking down lactic acid at the same speed as it is produced.

If the level of intensity increases further, and with it the share of anaerobic energy supply, the body's capacity to break down lactic acid is surpassed. Because of the accumulation of lactic acid and the fast depletion of carbohydrate stores, this type of exercise can be maintained for a limited period of time, which depends on the athlete's training status.

During maximal sprint training or highly intensive intervals, Type IIb fibers increase in importance. Energy supply during such activity is solely anaerobic, with carbohydrates serving as the fuel. These workouts result in very high lactate values, and thus the duration of exercise is short. Tables 1.5 through 1.8 further compare the characteristics of the muscle fibers. Graph 8 compares contraction power of fast and slow muscle fibers.

Table 1.5 Muscle Fiber Type, Duration of Exercise, Energy System, and Sports Activity

Muscle fibers	Duration	Energy system	Sports activities
FT fibers, Type II	Less than 30 sec	ATP and CP	Throwing and jumping,100-m sprint, tennis, baseball
FT and ST fibers, Type IIb	30 sec to 1 min	ATP-CP + Lactate system	200- to 400-m sprint, 100-m swimming, 500-m speedskating
ST and FT fibers, Type IIa	1.5-3 min	Lactate system, oxygen system	800-m running, boxing @ 3 min/round, wrestling, 1,500-m speedskating
ST fibers, Type I	More than 3 min	Oxygen system	Marathon, cross-country running and skiing, cycling

Note: FT= Fast twitch; ST= Slow twitch

Table 1.6 Characteristics of Red and White Muscle Fibers

White or fast Type II fibers (fast twitch)	Red or slow Type I fibers (slow twitch)
Explosiveness/sprinting capacity	Endurance capacity
Moderately capillaried	Well capillaried
Large anaerobic capacity	Large aerobic capacity
Small aerobic capacity	Small anaerobic capacity
Energy supply: Lactate system, direct ATP/CP	Energy supply: oxygen system
No increase of white fibers by training	Increase of red fibers by training
Duration: short	Duration: long
Lactate production: high	Lactate production: none
Age: decrease in white fibers	Age: no decrease in red fibers
Easily tired	Not easily tired
Speed: high	Speed: low
Contraction power: great	Contraction power: small

Table 1.7 Characteristics of Type I, Type IIa, and Type IIb Fibers

	Type I	Type IIa	Type IIb
Energy supply	Aerobic	Aerobic–anaerobic	Anaerobic
Fuel	Fats	Carbohydrates & fats	Carbohydrates
Exercise	Light	Intermediate	Heavy
Duration	Long (hours)	Intermediate (1-2 h)	Short
Lactate production	None	Moderate	High
Speed	Slow	Fast	High/maximum

Table 1.8 Type of Fiber and Intensity of Exercise

Intensity of exercise	Active fibers	Fuel
Light	Type I	Fats
Intermediate	Type I + IIa	Fats, carbohydrates
Heavy	Type I + Type IIa + IIb	Carbohydrates

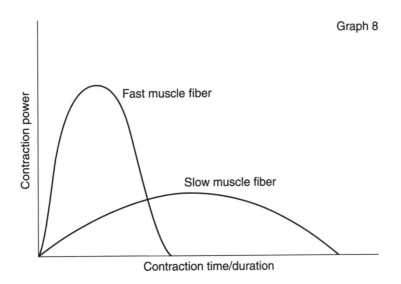

Graph 8

Targeted Training
==================

The principles of energy supply and the three energy-supplying systems—
the phosphate system, the lactate system, and the oxygen system—have
been described. Next is a discussion of how important these energy-supplying systems are for all types of sport. Effective training that leads to
maximum achievement is only possible when the principles of energy
supply are well understood and applied.

Every sport has its own specific training methods. A marathon runner's
training will be different from that of a sprinter. The marathon runner will
profit greatly by a large aerobic endurance capacity, so his or her training
should aim to improve the oxygen system to enlarge aerobic capacity. For the
sprinter, a maximum capacity of the phosphate system is essential, and so
training should aim to increase high-energy phosphates. Some sports, such
as middle-distance running, require training in all three energy-supplying
systems. Athletes who run the 400-meter, the 800-meter, and the 1,500-meter
need both a high aerobic capacity and a high anaerobic capacity. They must
learn how to fight the strong acidosis in their muscles and the accompanying
fatigue. In so doing they train their tolerance capacity.

The conclusion is that training should be aimed specifically at the energy
system involved in the sports activity. In other words, optimal training takes
place at a workout intensity that maximally activates the complete energy
system necessary for the sport. It is an art to assess training intensity correctly.
An intensity that is too low will not improve performance, but an intensity
that is too high may actually decrease performance and result in overtraining.
An important principle of training is that as the state of conditioning increases, the training stimulus, or intensity, should increase as well.

In summary, training should be specific, targeted at the energy system involved in the particular sport. Training intensity is essential for reaching maximum performance. As conditioning improves, training intensity should also increase, which means that training schemes should be continually evaluated and adapted. Figures 1.1 and 1.2 show the sources of energy needed for different types of training.

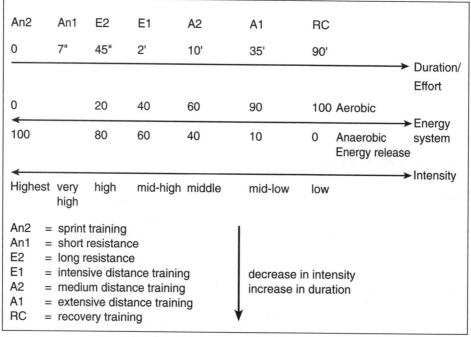

Figure 1.1   Energy system, duration, and intensity by training method.

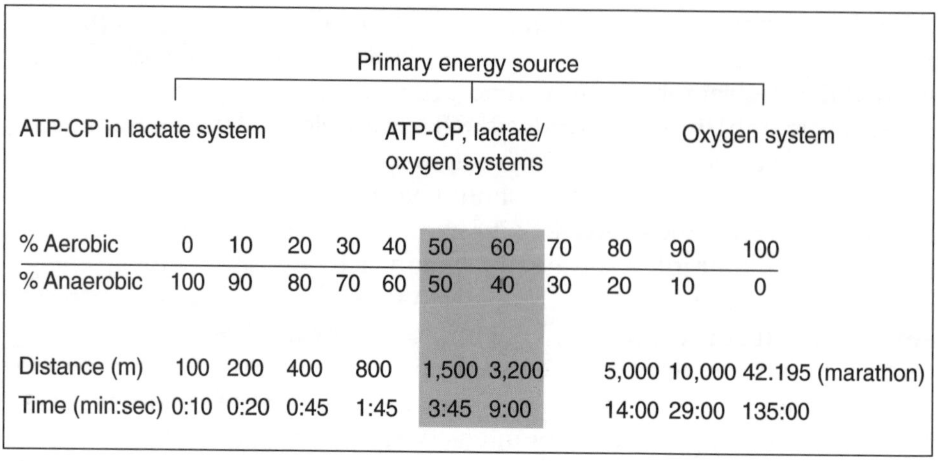

Figure 1.2   Primary energy sources of the most popular running distances.

In this book I have adopted the new international designations of the three intensity zones: the aerobic zone, the endurance zone, and the anaerobic zone. In the aerobic zone, energy supply comes from purely aerobic processes. The endurance zone is just under and just over the anaerobic threshold, so energy supply is partially aerobic and partially anaerobic. The anaerobic zone is based on energy supply without sufficient oxygen intake, which may lead to lactate accumulation.

The zones are as follows:

A1 = aerobic 1; the intensity is very low, about 70% to 80% of the anaerobic threshold

A2 = aerobic 2; the intensity is somewhat higher, 80% to 90% of the anaerobic threshold

E1 = endurance 1; in the transition zone, 90% to 100% of the anaerobic threshold

E2 = endurance 2; high-intensity endurance, 100% to 110% of the anaerobic threshold

An1 = anaerobic 1, based on anaerobic glycolysis, maximum energy supply 2 to 3 minutes

An2 = anaerobic 2, based on phosphates, maximum energy supply up to 10 seconds.

Table 1.9 compares the shares of the various energy systems used during different running events. The table shows that a marathon runner is supplied

Table 1.9 Running Events

	Marathon			
Distance	**Duration**	**Speed of phosphate system**	**Aerobic capacity: oxygen system**	**Anaerobic capacity: phosphate and lactate system**
42,195 m	130-180 min	0	95	5
10,000 m	28-50 min	5	80	15
5,000 m	14-26 min	10	70	20
3,000 m	9-16 min	20	40	40
1,500 m	4-6 min	20	25	55
800 m	2-3 min	30	5	65
400 m	1-1.5 min	80	5	15
200 m	0:22-0:35 sec	98	0	2
100 m	0:10-0:16 sec	98	0	2

Note: The relation between the duration of exercise and the percentage share of the various energy systems applies to every sport. The duration of the exercise determines the energy system that is used.

with 95% of aerobic energy and 5% of anaerobic energy. The table also can be used for events other than running events. For a swimming event that lasts 4 to 5 minutes, a comparable event is the 1,500 meter (with a running time of 4 to 6 minutes); the table shows that 20% of training should be targeted at improving the phosphate system (i.e., sprint workouts), 25% should be targeted at increasing aerobic endurance (oxygen system), and 55% should be targeted at improving anaerobic capacity (phosphate and lactate system). The duration of the exercise, in connection with intensity, determines the energy system that is used. Table 1.10 gives further examples of energy supply for various sports.

Training the Phosphate System

When training sprint capacity, the phosphate system is activated. So this training is anaerobic and alactic.

Sprints at maximum speed completely exhaust the store of high-energy phosphates after a few seconds. Sprinting capacity can best be trained by interval workouts with a great number of repetitions. In fact, sprint workouts are not really intervals because recovery is nearly complete. The intensity of the sprints can be both maximal and submaximal. At maximum speed the sprint takes some 6 to 8 seconds, submaximally 20 to 30 seconds. The key factor is the complete depletion of the high-energy phosphates without an accumulation of lactate. It takes about 6 seconds to reach maximum speed out of a standstill position, so the sprint has to be at least 50 to 60 meters. The pause between two sprints should be long enough to allow resynthesis of high-energy phosphates, ATP and CP; if pauses are too short, the lactate system will be activated. The duration of the pause should be 3 to 5 minutes, depending on the athlete's conditioning.

The recovery periods should include no exercise at all, because the store of ATP/CP resynthesizes more quickly during complete rest. Light exercise carried out during the recovery period partially blocks the replenishment of ATP/CP. This results in insufficient ATP/CP in store for the following sprint, so that the lactate system is also activated, bringing the undesirable side effect of lactate accumulation. HR monitoring is not suitable for directing and correcting sprint workouts, but lactate determination is appropriate. Graph 9 shows how ATP/CP levels differ depending on the type of recovery used.

Training the Lactate System

There are many forms of workout to train the lactate system. Tolerance training workouts are intensive. These forms of training are anaerobic and lactic. Whenever the distances of sprint workouts increase, the lactate system will be activated and the speed will become submaximal. The highest lactate levels occur in 400- to 800-meter races.

Intensive exercise lasting between 1 and 3 minutes activates and exhausts the lactate system to its maximum. Like the phosphate system, the lactate system can best be trained by interval workouts. The recovery periods

Table 1.10 Percentage Share in Total Energy Supply for Various Sports

Sport	Phosphate and lactate system	Lactate and oxygen system	Oxygen system
Baseball	80	20	—
Basketball	85	15	—
Field hockey	60	20	20
American football	90	10	—
European football	60	20	20
Golf	95	5	—
Gymnastics	90	10	—
Ice hockey	80	20	—
Rowing	20	30	50
Skiing			
Downhill, slalom	80	20	—
Cross-country	—	5	95
Recreational	34	33	33
Swimming			
50 m	98	2	—
100 m	80	15	5
200 m	30	65	5
400 m	20	40	40
800-1,500 m	10	20	70
Tennis	70	20	10
Track & field			
100-200 m	98	2	—
Throwing, jumping	90	10	—
400 m	80	15	5
800 m	30	65	5
1,500 m	20	55	25
3,000 m	20	40	40
5,000 m	10	20	70
10,000 m	5	15	80
Marathon	—	5	95
Volleyball	90	10	—
Cycling*			
Road races	—	5	95
Wrestling	90	10	—

*The share of anaerobic energy supply in cycling is only 5%. This by no means indicates that this source of energy is unimportant. On the contrary, in cycling the anaerobic factor is decisive. Being able to make the decisive escape, during 1-3 min, marks the difference between the winner and the rest of the pack.

Among other factors the capacity of the anaerobic systems determines whether a pro cyclist will be an elite racer. At the decisive moment, the top athlete can rely on a superior anaerobic capacity and make the final escape.

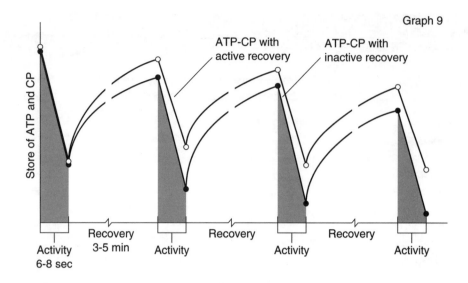

Graph 9

should not be so long that blood lactate concentrations decrease too much. This means that recovery periods, with an active recovery, should take 30 seconds to a few minutes, depending on the athlete's condition. The lactate system may best be trained with preparatory races. However, two very intensive races with high lactate values within 1 week might be too much. Such heavy exercise should always be followed by very light workouts, or recovery workouts. Graphs 10 and 11 show heart rates for repeated brief intense exercise followed by recovery.

Training the Oxygen System

The oxygen system can best be trained by means of endurance workouts, that is, exercise of relatively long duration at submaximal level. In endurance

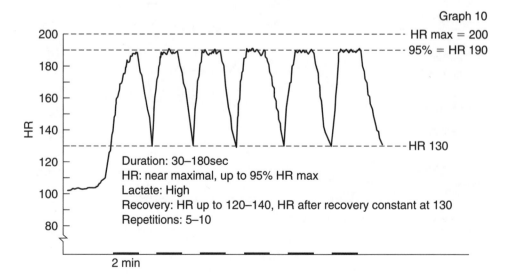

Graph 10

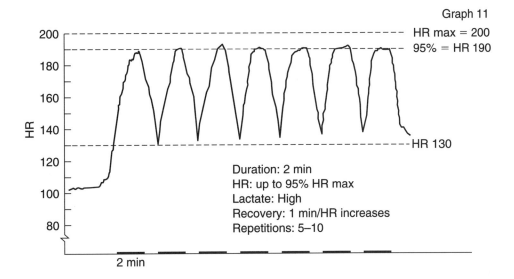

Graph 11

Duration: 2 min
HR: up to 95% HR max
Lactate: High
Recovery: 1 min/HR increases
Repetitions: 5–10

workouts there is no lactate accumulation. Endurance training takes place at different intensity levels, each of which should be trained in a specific way. There are four types of endurance workouts: intensive endurance training, intermediate endurance training, extensive endurance training, and the recovery workout.

Intensive Endurance Training

Short, intensive endurance training has a workload duration between 2 and 8 minutes and can best be achieved by interval workouts, as a rule at about 90% of maximum HR (HRmax). During this workout, the oxygen system is activated completely, and its intensity is slightly over or slightly under the deflection point. (The deflection point is described in chapter 3.) A small increase of lactate values up to 5 or 6 millimoles per liter is acceptable. This workout could be seen as an intermediate form between aerobic and anaerobic training. Recovery time is 4 to 6 minutes, and the number of repetitions is five to eight. This training workout should not be performed more often than twice a week. Graph 12 shows an example of intensive endurance training.

The longer intensive endurance workouts take 8 to 15 minutes, and these are also conducted in blocks, or intervals. Their intensity is a lactate value of about 3 and 4 millimoles per liter, which is 85% to 90% of HRmax. Recovery time is about 5 minutes. The number of repetitions is four to five, and the frequency is once or twice a week. These intensive endurance workouts are effective only when the athlete has rested sufficiently (see graph 13).

The athlete who notices fatigue in his or her legs should end this workout. If this type of workout is carried out despite fatigue and insufficient recovery, the chance of exhaustion and overtraining is considerable.

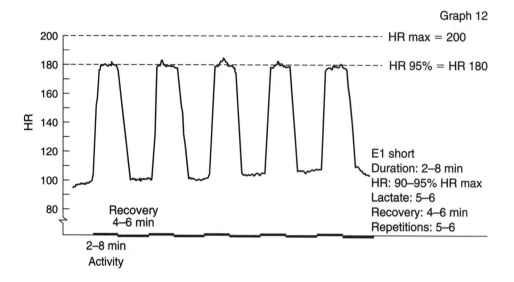

Graph 12

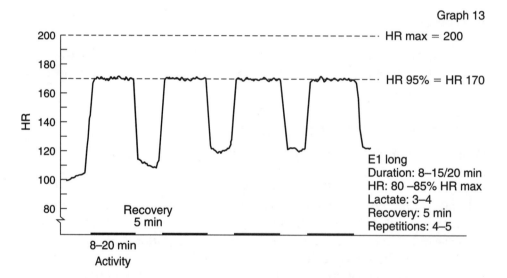

Graph 13

Intermediate Endurance Training

Intermediate endurance training workouts, such as the long rides of the cyclist and the long runs of the marathoner, are conducted at intermediate intensity. There is no lactate accumulation. Energy supply comes from the oxidation of fats and carbohydrates. HR range is between 80% and 85% of HRmax (see graph 14). The duration of these workouts depends on the duration of the race. As a rule, the race distance is surpassed once a week.

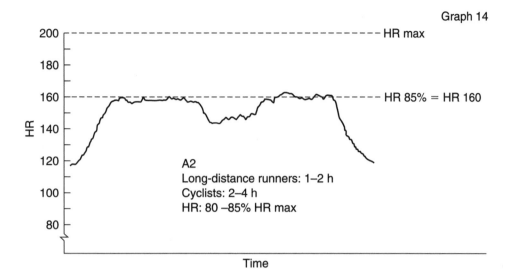

Graph 14

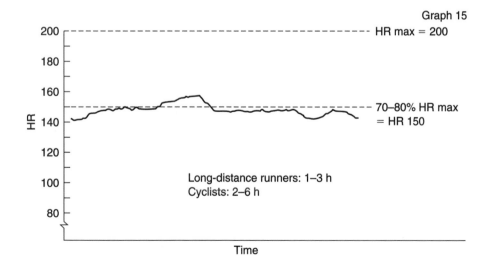

Extensive Endurance Training

These are the long, quiet endurance workouts: for the cyclist the rides of 100 to 200 kilometers, for the marathoner the 30-kilometer runs. HR range is between 70% and 80% of HRmax (see graph 15). Fat oxidation is optimal. Workouts for intermediate and extensive endurance training often are combined. These workouts are important because training the oxidation of fats saves carbohydrates longer, so that higher intensity exercise can be maintained longer.

Graph 15

Recovery Workouts

Recovery is an essential part of training. Very often light activity is better than complete rest. The intensity of recovery workouts is low, less than 70% of the HRmax. At this low intensity, aerobic capacity cannot be expected to improve (see graph 16).

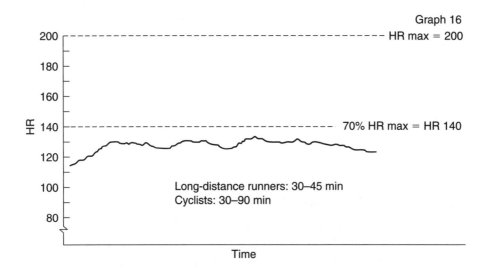

Graph 16

chapter 2

Heart Rate

In training practice, heart rate (HR) often is used as the standard for exercise intensity. There is a linear connection between HR and training intensity, as shown in graph 17 (page 26). Therefore, HR can be a good indicator of training intensity.

An optimal endurance training workout takes place at an intensity that activates the entire oxygen transport system. At this intensity there is no lactate accumulation. Therefore, this intensity range is called the aerobic/anaerobic transition zone.

In general, many of the so-called endurance workouts are done with an HR of about 180 beats per minute (bpm). For many athletes this HR is far above the aerobic/anaerobic transition zone. The aerobic/anaerobic transition zone may vary widely from person to person, but roughly this zone lies between 140 and 180 bpm.

Counting the Heart Rate

The best place to count HR is at the wrist (the wrist artery), the neck (the carotid artery), the temple (the temporal artery), or the left side of the chest. The morning pulse is always counted before getting out of bed, to ensure day-to-day consistency in the measurement. The data are plotted in a curve, as shown in graph 18.

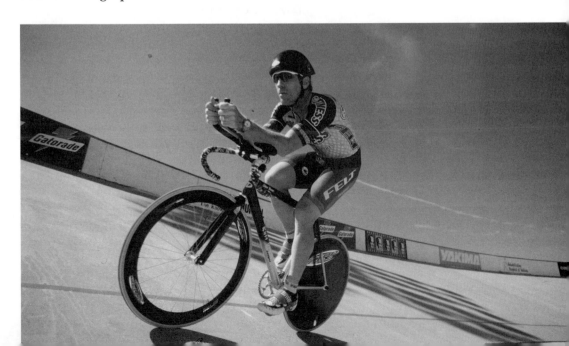

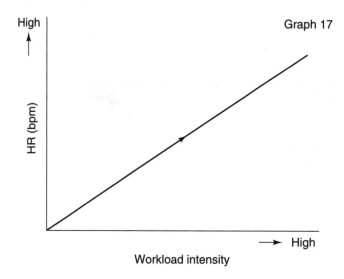

Graph 17

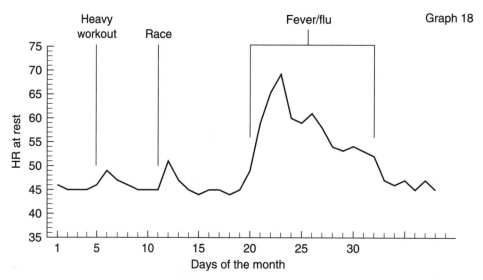

Graph 18

The 15-Beat Method

With this method, the athlete establishes the heartbeat and starts a stopwatch directly on a heartbeat. The athlete then starts counting at the next heartbeat and at the 15th heartbeat presses the stopwatch again. Suppose the time for 15 heartbeats is 20.3 seconds. The number of heartbeats per minute then is $(15 \div 20.3) \times 60 = 44$ bpm.

The 15-Second Counting Method

This method is easier but less accurate. The athlete counts heartbeats during 15 seconds and multiplies the number counted by four to get the number of heartbeats per minute. If 12 heartbeats are counted in 15 seconds, the HR is $4 \times 12 = 48$ bpm.

HR After Exercise

The exercise HR may best be counted by means of the 10-beat method. Immediately after exercise, the athlete uses a stopwatch to measure the time for 10 consecutive beats. The HR can be read in table 2.1.

The athlete presses the stopwatch at a beat (this is Beat 0) and counts to 10, pressing the stopwatch again at Beat 10. A disadvantage of this method is that HR decreases rapidly immediately after exercise stops. The HR obtained through this method will be slightly lower than the actual HR during exercise.

Table 2.1   Ten-Beat Method of Counting HR

Time (sec)	HR (bpm)	Time (sec)	HR (bpm)	Time (sec)	HR (bpm)
3.1	194	4.1	146	5.1	118
3.2	188	4.2	143	5.2	115
3.3	182	4.3	140	5.3	113
3.4	177	4.4	136	5.4	111
3.5	171	4.5	133	5.5	109
3.6	167	4.6	130	5.6	107
3.7	162	4.7	128	5.7	105
3.8	158	4.8	125	5.8	103
3.9	154	4.9	122	5.9	102
4.0	150	5.0	120	6.0	100

Maximum Heart Rate

The untrained athlete depicted in graph 19 (page 28) has a maximum heart rate (HRmax) of 200 bpm. After a period of endurance training this HRmax remains the same, so HRmax does not depend on the athlete's state of conditioning. In very well-trained athletes, HRmax might decrease slightly with training.

It is difficult to establish HRmax without technical aids. During maximum effort it is impossible to count one's HR. Counting immediately after the maximum effort will yield an inaccurate result, because HR decreases greatly immediately after exercise stops. HRmax may be roughly estimated based on age, according to the following formula:

$$HRmax = 220 - age$$

According to this formula, a 30-year-old person has an HRmax of 190 bpm. This formula is only a rough estimation and is not always accurate.

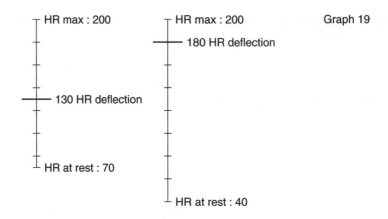

20 years old/untrained
HR 70–130 = Aerobic energy supply
HR 130–200 = Anaerobic energy supply

After training period
HR 40–180 = Aerobic energy supply
HR 180–200 = Anaerobic energy supply

Determining HRmax

HRmax can be reached only if the athlete has rested well enough. A complete recovery after the last workout is essential. To determine HRmax, the athlete starts with a warm-up, a period of light running or riding, followed by an intensive ride or run of 4 to 5 minutes. The last 20 to 30 seconds consists of an all-out sprint. HRmax now can be read easily using an HR monitor. Counting the pulse immediately after the effort is inaccurate, because of mistakes and because of the fast decrease in HR immediately after the effort.

HRmax should not be based on one recording but rather on several recordings taken over a few weeks. The highest value attained is the real HRmax. A very well-trained athlete may have an HRmax that is somewhat lower than that of a less well-trained person.

In the same person, HRmax may vary widely for different sports. One athlete may reach an HRmax of 203 while running but 187 when cycling. Athletes who are active in various sports are advised to establish their sport-specific HRmax. Training programs then can be developed on the basis of HRmax and the resting HR (HRrest).

Accurately counting HR is a fairly unreliable method, more so during an effort, but HR monitors have solved this problem. Every heartbeat—from HRrest to HRmax—may be read out directly. The most sophisticated HR monitors have a memory function, enabling the athlete to print out the HR curve after every training workout or race.

Heart Rate at Rest

In well-trained endurance athletes, the HRrest is very low. In untrained persons, HRrest is between 70 and 80 bpm. As endurance capacity is improved, HRrest gradually decreases. In well-trained endurance athletes (such as cyclists and marathoners), HRrest may be 40 to 50 bpm, or in some cases even lower.

In women, the HRrest is about 10 beats higher than in men of the same age. In the morning, the HRrest is about 10 beats lower than that in the evening for most people. But some have a lower evening HR than morning HR.

It is a widespread but erroneous belief that the lower the morning pulse, the better the condition. Conclusions about condition cannot be drawn from a low morning pulse. More important is the information the HRrest gives about recovery from a workout or race. Overtraining can be traced at an early stage by measuring the morning pulse, as can all kinds of viral infections (e.g., colds, and flu). The morning pulse increases in cases of overtraining and infections, whereas it gradually decreases as the athlete's condition improves. Every athlete who is serious about sport should draw up an HR curve similar to graph 20.

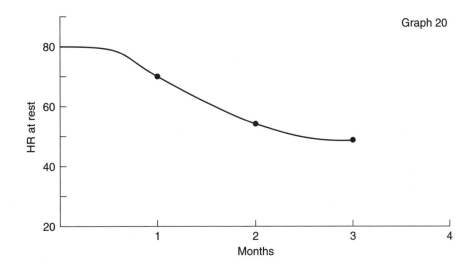

Graph 20

HR and Training Intensity

The method of the maximal HR reserve was developed by the Finnish scientist J. Karvonen. The HR reserve is the difference between HRmax and HRrest.

$$HR\ reserve = HRmax - HRrest$$

For an athlete who has an HRrest of 65 and an HRmax of 200, the HR reserve is $200 - 65 = 135$. The target HR (HRtarget) is then determined by adding a certain percentage of the HR reserve to HRrest. The HRtarget of 70% of the HR reserve is calculated as follows:

$$HRtarget = HRrest + 70\%\ of\ HR\ reserve$$

$$HRtarget = 65 + (0.7 \times 135) = 65 + 95 = 160\ bpm$$

See table 2.2 for training intensities formulated by the method of Karvonen.

Table 2.2 Training Intensities

Training Recovery		A1		A2		E1		E2		An1	
HR rest 40	60	40	60	40	60	40	60	40	60	40	60
Intensity 60%	60%	70%	70%	80%	80%	85%	85%	90%	90%	95%	95%
HR max											
210 142	150	159	165	176	180	185	188	193	195	202	203
208 141	149	158	164	174	178	183	186	191	193	200	201
206 140	148	156	162	173	177	181	184	189	191	198	199
204 138	146	155	161	171	175	179	182	188	190	196	197
202 137	145	153	159	170	174	178	181	186	188	194	195
200 136	144	152	158	168	172	176	179	184	186	192	193
198 135	143	151	157	166	170	174	177	182	184	190	191
196 134	142	149	155	165	169	173	176	180	182	188	189
194 132	140	148	154	163	167	171	174	179	181	186	187
192 131	139	146	152	162	166	169	172	177	179	184	185
190 130	138	145	151	160	164	168	171	175	177	183	184
188 129	137	144	150	158	162	166	169	173	175	181	182
186 128	136	142	148	157	161	164	167	171	173	179	180
184 126	134	141	147	155	159	162	165	170	172	177	178
182 125	133	139	145	154	158	161	164	168	170	175	176
180 124	132	138	144	152	156	159	162	166	168	173	174
178 123	131	137	143	150	154	157	160	164	166	171	172
176 122	130	135	141	149	153	156	159	162	164	169	170
174 120	128	134	140	147	151	154	157	161	163	167	168
172 119	127	132	138	146	150	152	155	159	161	165	166
170 118	126	131	137	144	148	151	154	157	159	164	165
168 117	125	130	136	142	146	149	152	155	157	162	163
166 116	124	128	134	141	145	147	150	153	155	160	161
164 114	122	127	133	139	143	145	148	152	154	158	159
162 113	121	125	131	138	142	144	147	150	152	156	157
160 112	120	124	130	136	140	142	145	148	150	154	155
158 111	119	123	129	134	138	140	143	146	148	152	153
156 110	118	121	127	133	137	139	142	144	146	150	151
154 108	116	120	126	131	135	137	140	143	145	148	149
152 107	115	118	124	130	134	135	138	141	143	146	147
150 106	114	117	123	128	132	134	137	139	141	145	146
148 105	113	116	122	126	130	132	135	137	139	143	144
146 104	112	114	120	125	129	130	133	135	137	141	142
144 102	110	113	119	123	127	128	131	134	136	139	140
142 101	109	111	117	122	126	127	130	132	134	137	138
140 100	108	110	116	120	124	125	128	130	132	135	136

Two athletes running at the same pace may reach different HRs. However, it may not be correct to conclude that the athlete who reaches the higher HR is doing a heavier workout. For example, one runner has an HRmax of 210 bpm, whereas the HR while running is 160 bpm. The other runner has an HRmax of 170 and reaches 140 bpm. The first runner performs at 50 beats under his or her maximum HR and the second at 30. In this example, the second runner is doing a heavier workout. Once the HRrest and the HRmax are known, the intensity of exercise can be assessed with another formula by Karvonen:

$$\frac{\text{HR during exercise} - \text{HRrest}}{\text{HRmax} - \text{HRrest}} \times 100\%$$

If the two runners of the preceding example have the same HRrest of 50 bpm, their percentage of workload is 69% and 75%, respectively. Karvonen's percentage is about 10% higher than the percentage of maximum oxygen consumption ($\dot{V}O_2$max). So Karvonen's percentage of 75% corresponds to 65% of $\dot{V}O_2$max (see figure 2.3).

The HRtarget is deduced from the HRmax by using the following formula:

$$\text{HRtarget} = 0.75 \times \text{HRmax}$$

With an HRmax of 200, HRtarget will be $0.75 \times 200 = 150$ bpm. HRtarget as a percentage of HR reserve and HRtarget as a percentage of HRmax are not equal, as shown in table 2.4.

HRrest	60%	70%	80%	90%	100% HFmax	
110	175					
105	170	185	195		220	
100	165	180	190	205	215	
95	160	175	185	200	210	
90	155	170	180	195	205	15
85	150	165	175	190	200	20
80	145	160	170	185	195	25
75	140	155	165	180	190	30 / 35
70	135	150	160	175	185	40 / 45
65	130	145	155	170	180	50 / 55
60	125	140	150	165	175	60 / 65
55	120	135	145	160	170	70 / 80
50	115	130	140	155	165	
45	110	125	135	150	160	
40	105	120	130	145	155	
35	100	115	125	140	150	
30		110	120	135	145	
				130	140	

Table 2.3 Karvonen's percentage.

Table 2.4 HR Target Percentages of HRreserve and HRmax

HRtarget	% HRreserve	% HRmax**
186	90	93
180	85	90
173	80	87
166	75	83
160	70	80
153	65	76
146	60	73

*HRrest = 65

**HRmax = 200

As the HRtarget decreases, the difference between the two methods is more distinct. A HRtarget of 60% of HR reserve or 73% of HRmax is considered a threshold value. A workout with a lower HR does not improve aerobic capacity, because the training stimulus is too weak. To improve aerobic endurance capacity, the HRtarget should be somewhere between 60% and 90% of HR reserve. See tables 2.5 and 2.6 for HRtarget and training intensities.

Deflection Point

The most important change arising from endurance training is a shift of the deflection point to a higher HR. As explained in more detail later, the relationship between HR and exercise intensity is not linear at higher intensity levels. At a high intensity, the line representing this relationship, which is straight at first, shows a marked bend. In other words, exercise

Table 2.5 HR Targets

Age	20-29	30-39	40-49	50-59	60-69
HRmax	190	185	180	170	160
Highest HRtarget 0.9 (HRmax − 75) + 75*	179	174	170	161	152
Lowest HRtarget 0.6 (HRmax − 75) + 75	144	141	138	132	126
Average HRtarget 0.75 (HRmax − 75) + 75	155	152	149	141	139

*HRrest = 75.

Table 2.6   Rough Indication of Training Intensities

Based on HRreserve	% of HRreserve
Very light workout/recovery workout	50-60
Light aerobic workout	60-70
Intensive aerobic workout	70-80
Anaerobic workout 80-90	
Maximum effort in races	90-100
Based on HRmax	**% of HRmax**
Very light workout/recovery workout	68-73
Light aerobic workout	73-80
Intensive aerobic workout	80-87
Anaerobic workout 87-93	
Maximum effort in races	93-100

intensity can be increased but the athlete's HR lags behind from a certain point. This point is the HR deflection point (HRdefl). For example, an untrained person has an HRdefl of 130. After a period of endurance training, the HRdefl shifts from 130 to 180 bpm.

Any exercise with an intensity above the HRdefl will result in an accumulation of lactate. In well-trained endurance athletes, the HR range within which energy is supplied aerobically has increased enormously. This wider HR range corresponds with a large aerobic capacity, with which an endurance effort can be maintained long and at a high pace. An athlete with such an aerobic capacity is said to have stamina. Only during efforts of a very high intensity is the anaerobic system called on, with the formation of lactate as an unpleasant side effect.

Lactate Curve

The relationship between HR and lactate levels, known as the HR–lactate curve, varies among people, and it can vary within a person as his condition changes. In graph 21, the left-hand curve is one of an untrained person, whose HRdefl is at 130 bpm. The right-hand curve shows that after a period of training, the HRdefl has shifted to 180 bpm.

The untrained person can maintain an effort at an HR of 130 for a long period of time. The trained athlete can perform for a long period at an HR of 180. This intensity of effort corresponds with a lactate level of 4 millimoles per liter. This limit is also called the anaerobic threshold. An effort above the anaerobic threshold results in a steep increase of lactate.

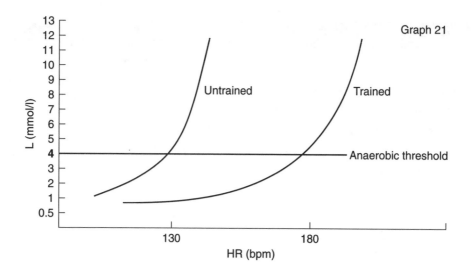

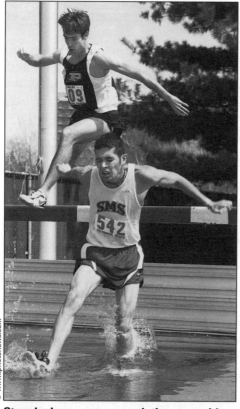

Steeplechase runners push the anaerobic threshold.

$\dot{V}O_2max$

The $\dot{V}O_2max$ is the maximal oxygen consumption during maximal effort lasting longer than 2 minutes and shorter than 5 minutes. $\dot{V}O_2max$ is expressed in liters per minute. During exercise at the level of $\dot{V}O_2max$, energy supply is both aerobic and anaerobic. Because anaerobic energy supply is limited, the athlete will have to decrease the exercise intensity after a short time.

Therefore, an endurance effort is done at an intensity less than the $\dot{V}O_2max$. Training increases the $\dot{V}O_2max$, but it is of far greater importance that training shifts the anaerobic threshold. After a few months of training, the anaerobic threshold may increase from 40% to 65% of the $\dot{V}O_2max$. That means that, influenced by training, lactate will only be formed at an intensity corresponding to a higher percentage of the $\dot{V}O_2max$. To put it more simply, the pace may increase greatly before acidosis takes place. So training increases the $\dot{V}O_2max$ but, even more important, it increases the percentage of the $\dot{V}O_2max$ at which exercise can be maintained for a long period of time.

The right-hand vertical axis of graph 22 shows the shift of the HRdefl after a training period. Untrained, the HRdefl is at 130 bpm. After a few months of training, the HRdefl increases to 180 bpm. The left-hand vertical axis shows the $\dot{V}O_2$max increase, especially the increase in the percentage of $\dot{V}O_2$max at which exercise can be maintained for a long period of time. Through training, the $\dot{V}O_2$max may improve up to 30% (see graph 23). Table 2.7 shows the relationship between HRmax and $\dot{V}O_2$max.

Because training workouts at $\dot{V}O_2$max can be maintained only about 5 minutes, $\dot{V}O_2$max is not a suitable standard for the endurance athlete's performance capacity. A better standard is the anaerobic or lactate threshold.

This anaerobic or lactate threshold corresponds to the maximum level of exercise that an athlete can maintain for a long period of time without accumulation of lactate. After a period of endurance training, there is a considerable change in HR with the same workload.

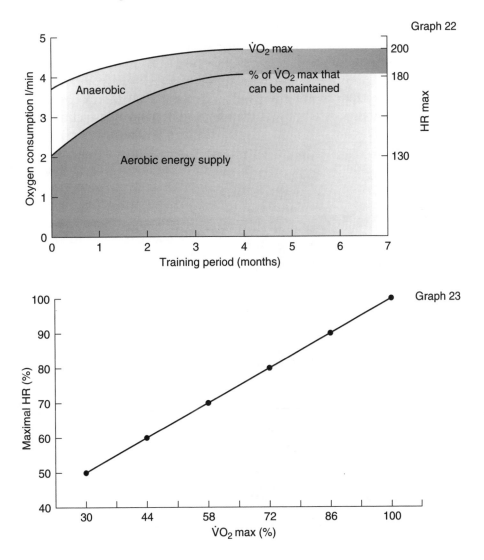

Graph 22

Graph 23

Table 2.7 Relation between HRmax and $\dot{V}O_2$max	
Percentage of HRmax	**Percentage of $\dot{V}O_2$ max**
50	30
60	44
70	58
80	72
90	86
100	100

Conconi's Method

This book was prompted by the world hour record that cyclist Francesco Moser (Italy) set in January 1984 in Mexico City. Moser improved the record set by Eddy Merckx (Belgium) in October 1972, also in Mexico City. Eddy Merckx, called "the cannibal" because he won every race, was pronounced the best cyclist of the 20th century long before the year 2000. Merckx has always said that the 1 hour in Mexico was the toughest of his whole cycling career.

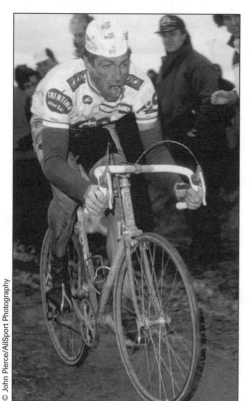

In two attempts, one after the other, Moser rode as much as 1,719 meters more than Merckx. Reaching 51.151 kilometers, Moser was the first cyclist to break the magic limit of 50 kilometers. Another record was set that was expected to stand for decades.

Exercise Intensity and HR

In formulating the method that bears his name, sports physiology professor Francesco Conconi of the Ferrara University (Italy) used the existing relationship between exercise intensity and HR. Like scientists in the past, he found that the relationship between HR and exercise intensity was no longer linear at higher intensity levels. At a high intensity, the line representing this relationship,

© John Pierce/AllSport Photography

Record-breaker Italian Francesco Moser.

which is straight at first, shows a marked bend. In other words, exercise intensity can be increased but the athlete's HR lags behind from a certain point. This point is the HRdefl. The exercise intensity corresponding to this point is the maximum effort that is purely supplied by aerobic energy. The bend in the curve indicates at what HR or what exercise intensity (e.g., the pace of running or cycling) the body shifts from mainly aerobic energy to mainly anaerobic energy supply. With this knowledge, Conconi was able to indicate exactly at what speed Moser had to cycle in his record attempt without premature exhaustion.

The bend in graph 24 indicates the maximum speed that corresponds with the HRdefl; this speed can be maintained for a long period of time. It is the highest speed that is completely supplied by aerobic energy. If this speed should be increased beyond the HRdefl, lactate will begin to accumulate. At this higher speed, the aerobic energy supplying system fails. The anaerobic system springs into action, resulting in the ever-increasing lactate accumulation.

A big advantage of Conconi's method is that there is no need of a blood sample, which is why it is also called the noninvasive method for determining the HRdefl. Conconi's method will be amply dealt with later in this book.

The Merckx–Moser era seems to be ages behind us now. The current records are claimed by riders like Graeme Obree (Scotland), Miguel Indurain (Spain), Tony Rominger (Switzerland), and Chris Boardman (England).

As mentioned, Moser was coached at the time by Conconi, whose method of determining HR and exercise intensity was the basis of Moser's success and also was a breakthrough in sports medicine and training. Tony Rominger was coached by Dr. Michele Ferrari, one of Conconi's former pupils. Ferrari works with the same principles with which Conconi and Moser introduced the new era in 1972.

Although such breakthroughs in sports medicine and training are very important, sports medicine alone never determines whether a record will be

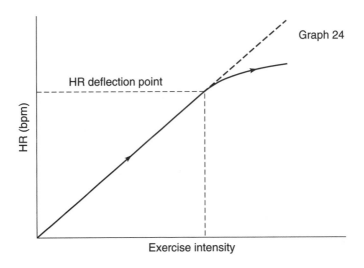

Graph 24

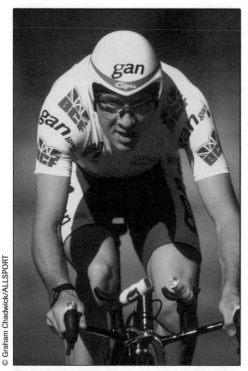

Chris Boardman set a new record, covering 56 kilometers in one hour.

broken. The key factor is the athlete's talent; without sufficient talent, a world record will never be possible. But with talent alone the absolute top will not be reached either, because talent must be developed to its maximum. In that respect, Italian sport science is far ahead of the rest of the world of cycling. Sports medicine and coaching are optimal in Italy, with the logical results. The gap between riders coached in Italy and the rest of the world seems nearly unbridgeable.

On November 5, 1994, Rominger wrote a new chapter in the history of cycling. On the wooden track of Bordeaux, he rode 55.291 kilometers in 1 hour. Exactly 6,129.8 times he turned his giant gear of 9.02 meters around, 102.2 times every minute. This was exactly the same frequency with which Guiseppe Olmo cycled into legend in 1935 when he was the first to break the 45-kilometer limit. With 7.32 meters, Olmo then made 1.70 meters less per revolution than Rominger.

In that 1 hour, Rominger rode 5,860 meters more than Merckx. On the track in Bordeaux, 250 meters long, Merckx would have been overtaken 23 times. But Rominger's record did not hold very long. On September 6, 1996, Chris Boardman smashed the old record by 1,084 meters, covering 56.375 kilometers in 1 hour.

Pedaling Frequency

If we look at the development of the world hour record, it is striking that the pedaling frequency remains fairly constant. On the other hand, the gear has increased enormously. In other words, strength has increased tremendously with a constant frequency. Cyclists call this power. In other words, power = frequency + muscular strength.

It is a standing rule that the world hour record can be broken only when the rider can maintain a pedaling frequency between 100 and 105. As shown in table 2.8, the Scottish rider Obree is an exception to this rule, but he had a very different type of bike.

In September 2000, the International Cycling Union (UCI) decided to recognize Eddy Merckx's world hour record, achieved in Mexico City in 1972, as the official world record. That record was set on a normal racing bike with spoked wheels, without an aerodynamic helmet and in a classic cycling

Table 2.8 Gear and Pedaling Frequency of the World Hour Record

Year	Name	Place	Gain (m)	Dist. (m)	Gear	Freq.
1893	Desgrange (Fr)	Paris		35,325		
1894	Dubois (Fr)	Paris	2,895	38,220		
1897	Van den Eynde (Bel)	Paris	1,020	39,240		
1898	Hamilton (USA)	Denver	1,541	40,781		
1905	Petit-Breton (Fr)	Paris	329	41,110		
1907	Berthet (Fr)	Paris	410	41,520		
1912	Egg (Swi)	Paris	840	42,360		
1913	Berthet (Fr)	Paris	381	42,741		
1913	Egg (Swi)	Paris	784	43,525		
1913	Berthet (Fr)	Paris	250	43,775		
1914	Egg (Swi)	Paris	427	44,247		
1933	Van Hout (NL)	Roermond	341	44,588		
1933	Richard (Fr)	St. Truiden	189	44,777		
1935	Olmo (It)	Milan	290	45,067		
1936	Richard (Fr)	Milan	308	45,375		
1937	Slaats (NL)	Milan	160	45,535	$24 \times 7 = 7.32$	103.6
1937	Archambaud (Fr)	Milan	280	45,817	$24 \times 7 = 7.32$	104.3
1942	Coppi (It)	Milan	31	45,848	$52 \times 15 = 7.40$	103.3
1956	Anquetil (Fr)	Milan	311	46,159	$52 \times 15 = 7.40$	103.9
1956	Baldini (It)	Milan	234	46,393	$52 \times 15 = 7.40$	104.4
1957	Riviere (Fr)	Milan	530	46,923	$52 \times 15 = 7.40$	105.7
1958	Riviere (Fr)	Milan	423	47,346	$53 \times 15 = 7.54$	104.6
1967	Bracke (Bel)	Rome	747	48,093	$53 \times 15 = 7.54$	106.3
1968	Ritter (Den)	Mexico City	560	48,653	$54 \times 15 = 7.69$	105.4
1972	Merckx (Bel)	Mexico City	778	49,431	$52 \times 14 = 7.93$	103.9
1984	Moser (It)	Mexico City	1,377	50,808	$56 \times 15 = 8.17$	103.6
1984	Moser (It)	Mexico City	343	51,151	$57 \times 15 = 8.27$	103.0
1993	Obree (GB)	Hamar	445	51,596	$52 \times 12 = 9.25$	92.9
1993	Boardman (GB)	Bordeaux	674	52,270	$53 \times 13 = 8.70$	100.1
1994	Obree (GB)	Bordeaux	443	52,713	$52 \times 12 = 9.25$	94.9
1994	Indurain (Sp)	Bordeaux	327	53,040	$59 \times 14 = 8.86$	100.9
1994	Rominger (Swi)	Bordeaux	792	53,832	$59 \times 14 = 8.86$	101.3
1994	Rominger (Swi)	Bordeaux	1,459	55,291	$60 \times 14 = 9.02$	102.2
1996	Boardman (GB)	Manchester	1,084	56,375	$56 \times 13 = 9.02$	104.2

outfit. All the records set after Merckxs acheivment were deleted from the list, because of the aerodynamic gadgets used. There are rumors that the UCI wants to delete these records not only because of aerodynamics but also because erythropoietin and blood transfusions may have played a role.

The world hour record for women was in the hands of the Australian Anna Wilson on October 18, 2000, when she rode 43.500 kilometers on the new cycling track in Melbourne. The Frenchwoman Janine Longo broke that record on November 5, 2000, in Mexico City, the record on a traditional bike. She reached a distance of 44.767 kilometers, 1,267 meters more than Wilson did on October 18. In 1996, Longo had ridden 48.150 kilometers at an altitude of 2,000 meters in Mexico City, using an aerodynamic bike with solid wheels and pointed handlebars. The UCI decided in 2000 to recognize only those records set on normal bikes with spoked wheels, so Longo's time in Mexico City in 2000 stands as the world record for women.

Chris Boardman broke Eddy Merckx's record on October 27, 2000, in Manchester on a traditional bike with spokes. The Englishman reached a distance of 49.441 kilometers, exactly 10 meters more than Merckx did in Mexico City in 1972. So Boardman now holds the world hour record on a traditional bike and the unofficial record on a futuristic racing bike.

Cycling speed is determined by the gear and the frequency. The gear that a cyclist can handle depends on many factors:

- Power of the rider
- Weather conditions (front wind or tail wind)
- Road conditions (flat or uphill)
- Material
- Road surface (cobblestones or asphalt)

Efficient pedaling involves contracting the right muscles at the right time in the most economical way. Energy consumption should be as low as possible. Too big or too small a gear consumes extra energy and will decrease speed. In general, cyclists tend to use a gear that is too big. For every speed, there is an optimal pedaling frequency. This frequency is around 80 to 90 rotations per minute (RPM) for riding in a pack. In time trials and world hour records, this frequency is between 100 and 106 RPM. In long ascents in the Tour de France, the top climbers achieve 80 to 100 RPM. See graph 25.

A high frequency of rotations per minute has a number of undeniable advantages. When the muscles in the leg contract, the blood vessels in the leg are compressed. Then the blood is pressed out of the leg muscles in the direction of the heart. This mechanism is called the muscle pump of the legs. During the relaxing phase of the muscles, fresh blood flows into the muscle. During cycling, the athlete constantly alternates between contracting and relaxing leg muscles. With a bigger gear, the contraction phase is longer. The bigger the gear, the sooner oxygen is depleted and lactate begins to accumulate, resulting in

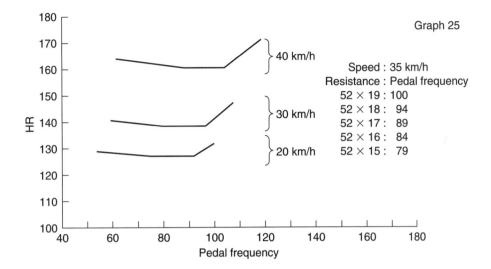

Graph 25

Speed : 35 km/h
Resistance : Pedal frequency
52 × 19 : 100
52 × 18 : 94
52 × 17 : 89
52 × 16 : 84
52 × 15 : 79

muscle soreness. In general, a high frequency is less tiring. Also, while riding with a smaller gear, the rider can react faster to changes in the pace and escapes.

Using a high frequency has an additional advantage. In triathlons, a running event follows the cycling event. The athlete who rides with a higher frequency will reach a higher leg cadence in running sooner and more easily. There is a relationship between optimal pedaling frequency and HRmax. The formula is 2 × pedaling frequency = HRmax. This formula may explain why older riders often use a bigger gear: As the athlete ages, the HRmax gradually decreases.

Cycling with a high frequency should be trained specifically; however, this is one of the poorly developed aspects of cycling training. For top achievement, the rider must train regularly at frequencies far above 100 RPM. In other words, the ability to ride with a high frequency is one of the decisive factors for optimal cycling.

If a cyclist trains on an ergometer with a constant workload (e.g., 300 watts) but at different frequencies, the differences between workouts are enormous. With the low frequency, the rider will feel sore leg muscles. With higher frequencies, breathing will become more difficult. So a high frequency especially burdens the cardiovascular system, and lower frequencies use muscular strength.

The training stimulus changes with varying frequencies and a constant workload. In other words, a workout with a frequency of 60 RPM at 300 watts is mainly a weight-training workout. The same load at 300 watts and a frequency of 100 RPM trains the cardiovascular system. Graph 26 shows the relationship between workload and frequency.

What does this mean for everyday practice on the road? When two cyclists ride side by side at the same pace but with a different gear—one rider with

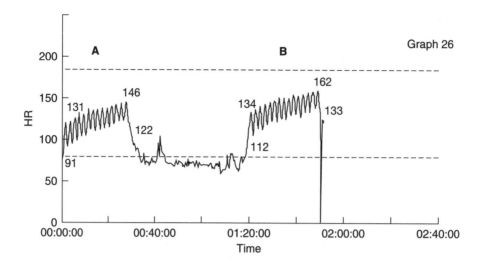

a low and the other with a high pedaling frequency—the rider with the big gear will mainly train muscular strength and the one with the small gear will mainly train the cardiovascular system. When the pace is increased, the first rider will fall behind because of fatigue in the leg and the second will fall behind because of shortness of breath.

Factors Influencing Heart Rate

Many factors can influence HR. Athletes and coaches must account for these factors in planning training and competitions.

Age

With age, HRmax gradually decreases. This decrease does not correlate with the state of conditioning. A 20-year-old may reach an HRmax of 220 bpm. At the age of 40, the HRmax is often no more than 180 bpm. There are fairly large differences in HRmax between people of the same age. One 40-year-old athlete may have a maximum of around 165, whereas another reaches an HRmax of 185.

As age increases, there is a linear decrease in HRmax, as shown in graphs 27 and 28.

$$HRmax = 220 - age$$

For a 40-year-old athlete this means:

$$HRmax = 220 - 40 = 180$$

Although there are many exceptions to this rule, it is a reasonably general rule; but it is inappropriate for athletes who wish to train on the basis of HR.

Not only does the HRmax decrease linearly with age, but also the HRrest and the HRdefl, the anaerobic threshold, follow the same line. The vertical bars in graph 27 mark possible differences between individuals of the same age.

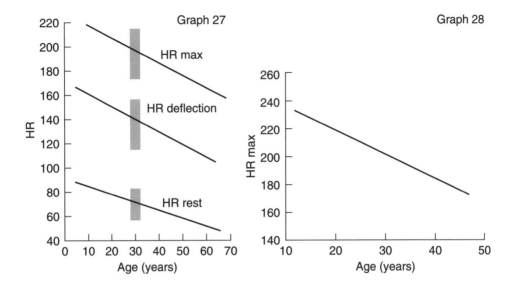

Graph 27

Graph 28

Graph 29 (page 44) depicts a running workout during which the HR is largely around 160. In a laboratory test on a bicycle ergometer, this triathlete reached an HRmax of 187 bpm. His calculated HRdefl was 160 bpm. So for a 42-year-old, this athlete has a rather high HRmax.

The first part of the run, up to about 50 minutes, is less than optimal, because the athlete doesn't reach the established HRdefl of 160. The intensity of the run between the 50th and the 150th minute is optimal, because the athlete's HR is always very close to the HRdefl. By the end of the run this athlete seems to have some energy left, because he is capable of running above the HRdefl for some time. The calculated HRdefl was determined in a sport-specific test. This will be treated in more detail in chapter 4.

Graph 30 (page 44) represents a runner whose HRmax, as determined by a sport-specific test, is 167 bpm. The calculated HRdefl is 142. In contrast with the previous athlete (represented in graph 29), this marathon runner has a rather low HRmax for his age. The HRdefl calculated for him is also considerably lower. He has done an excellent endurance workout with an HR always close to 140 bpm. So he runs just below his HRdefl.

The details of these two well-trained athletes show how big the difference in HRmax may be between two people of the same age. The triathlete will have to train his or her endurance capacity at an HR completely different from that of the marathoner.

Overtraining, Insufficient Recovery, and Illness

Depending on the type of overtraining, the morning pulse may be higher or extremely low. A morning pulse as low as 25 bpm is no exception. Normally during exercise, HR increases very rapidly to maximal values, but in a case of overtraining, HR may lag with high-intensity exercise. Also, with overtraining, HRmax is no longer attainable. So overtraining results in a completely different

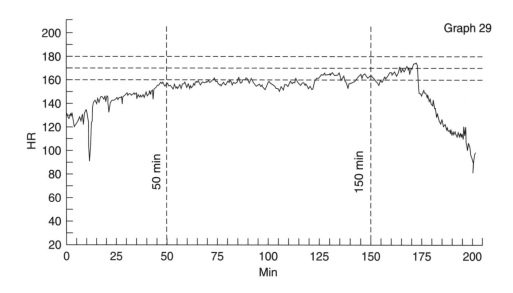

Graph 29

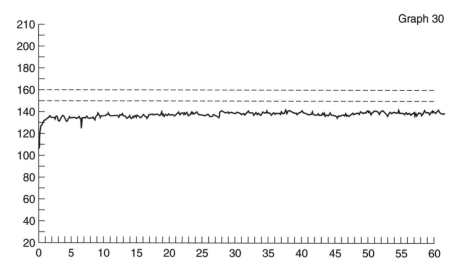

Graph 30

HR pattern, both at rest and during exercise. Constant HR measurements will indicate that something is wrong and that extra rest might make more sense than another heavy workout. With insufficient recovery, or during illness or convalescence, the HR curve shows a different pattern (see also chapter 5, Overtraining). Graph 31 shows that with insufficient recovery after an infectious disease, performance is distinctly diminished. During exercise, HR increases faster than under normal conditions with a relatively low pace.

Graph 32 shows that the athlete's condition has improved enormously. Thus, it only makes sense to train or race after complete recovery from an infectious disease. As shown in graph 31, premature return to training does more harm than good. It would have been better for this athlete to rest instead of race, or to perform a light workout at most.

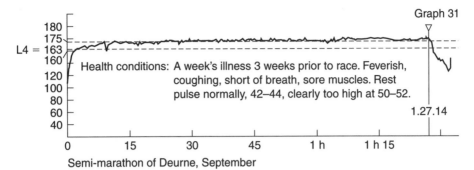

Graph 31

Health conditions: A week's illness 3 weeks prior to race. Feverish, coughing, short of breath, sore muscles. Rest pulse normally, 42–44, clearly too high at 50–52.

1.27.14

Semi-marathon of Deurne, September

Test data: Lactate 2 = HR 155; HR max = 180
           Lactate 3 = HR 160
           Lactate 4 = HR 163
Race: Not an easy run. A relatively high HR
      of 175 increasing with slower pace
Time: 1.27.14
Poor recovery after race.

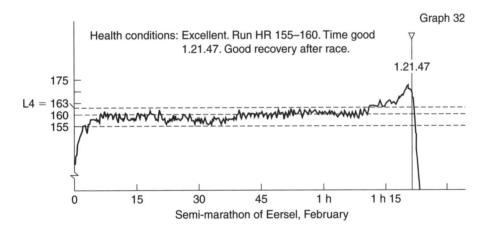

Graph 32

Health conditions: Excellent. Run HR 155–160. Time good 1.21.47. Good recovery after race.

1.21.47

Semi-marathon of Eersel, February

When an athlete is fully rested, the various HR levels—HRmax, HRdefl, and HRrest—are fairly constant. The day after a heavy workout or race, the morning pulse can be higher, which indicates that the body has not sufficiently recovered. Other indications of insufficient recovery include reduced HRdefl and HRmax. In the presence of these indicators, it is advisable not to train heavily in order to give the body a chance to recover. There is never any gain in performing a heavy workout after insufficient recovery; not only will there be no improvement, but the level of performance capacity will even decrease. Graphs 33, 34, and 35 illustrate the effects of insufficient recovery. The cyclist depicted in graphs 33, 34 and 35 had recovered well before Races 1 and 3, and he felt good during the races, achieving a high HRmax in both races. Race 2 was performed after insufficient recovery. The cyclist experienced sore legs, and HRmax clearly was not attained.

The data for the Tour de France and the Netherlands championship team time trial at Dronten show a clear decrease of HRmax and HRdefl. During the

Tour de France, the complete pack is constantly in a state of overtraining or at least insufficient recovery, which is expressed in the HR curves (see graphs 200, 203 and 204 in chapter 9).

When the morning pulse is high and the HR corresponding to a normal endurance workout cannot be reached or only at great cost, the best solution is complete rest or a recovery workout.

A low HR, lower than 50 bpm, generally is believed to characterize the well-trained heart. This slow HR may be even more extreme in some endurance athletes. During sleep, HR values between 20 and 30 can be reached. The slow HR is a normal adaptation to extreme endurance training and is not dangerous.

But an extremely low HR also may indicate that the heart is ill. A low HR can be a sign of a cardiac disease, which could even be fatal. It is of major importance to distinguish between the two situations.

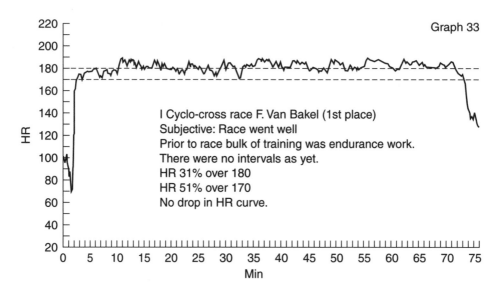

Graph 33

I Cyclo-cross race F. Van Bakel (1st place)
Subjective: Race went well
Prior to race bulk of training was endurance work.
There were no intervals as yet.
HR 31% over 180
HR 51% over 170
No drop in HR curve.

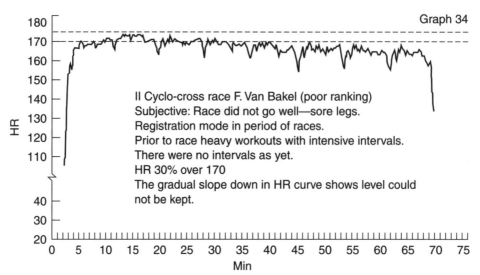

Graph 34

II Cyclo-cross race F. Van Bakel (poor ranking)
Subjective: Race did not go well—sore legs.
Registration mode in period of races.
Prior to race heavy workouts with intensive intervals.
There were no intervals as yet.
HR 30% over 170
The gradual slope down in HR curve shows level could not be kept.

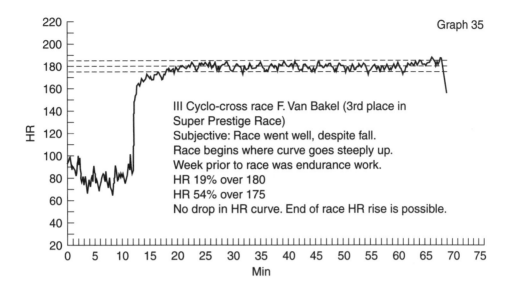

Graph 35

III Cyclo-cross race F. Van Bakel (3rd place in
Super Prestige Race)
Subjective: Race went well, despite fall.
Race begins where curve goes steeply up.
Week prior to race was endurance work.
HR 19% over 180
HR 54% over 175
No drop in HR curve. End of race HR rise is possible.

In case of a physiological adaptation, the stroke volume will compensate for the lower HR. If an athlete has no complaints and when tested shows an adequate increase in HR, there is certainly no need for aggressive treatment. But when the athlete complains about dizziness or fainting, matters should be investigated in more detail. There are examples of endurance athletes whose complaints about fainting were resolved only after they had stopped endurance training.

In extreme cases a pacemaker is required. These athletes are well advised to give up performance-oriented endurance sport, as well as sports like deep-sea diving, flying, and mountaineering.

Nutrition

Adequate nutrition can considerably improve performance in endurance sports, by as much as 7%. This improvement is expressed in a lower HR at an equal load. With a normal diet, the average HR during endurance sports is 156 ± 10 bpm. The average HR during endurance sports with 200 grams of carbohydrates is 145 ± 9 bpm (see graph 36).

Altitude

The first hours after an athlete arrives at a higher altitude, HRrest decreases, but then it increases. At 2,000 meters this increase is 10%, and at 4,500 meters it is 45%, starting from the individual HRrest at sea level. After some days, depending on the altitude, HR decreases again to normal values at rest or in many cases even falls below that value. Returning to the athlete's normal HRrest at a certain altitude indicates good acclimatization.

Because it is so easy to count HRrest, the degree of acclimatization can be established very simply. Any athlete who will stay at a high altitude for some time is advised to use the following simple method:

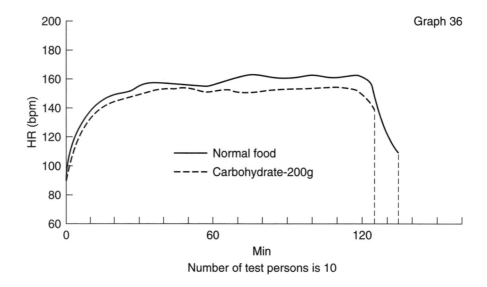

Graph 36

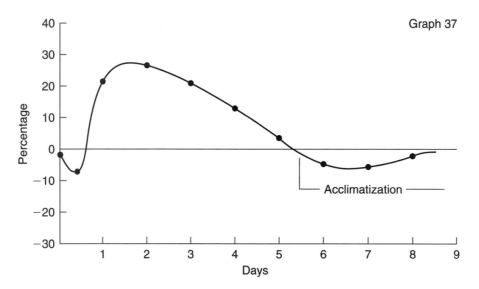

Graph 37

1. Take your morning pulse for some weeks before your departure, to establish your individual value.

2. During your stay at the new altitude, take your HR every day in the same way, to estimate the degree of acclimatization.

Graph 37 shows a plot of an athlete's acclimatization to altitude.

Medication

Various medications can affect HR. The best known are the beta-blockers, which are especially used for hypertension and angina pectoris. (Angina pectoris is a pain in the chest, mostly arising during physical exercise as a result of a stricture in a coronary artery.) Beta-blockers are known to decrease HRrest and HRmax, and they decrease endurance capacity by about 10%.

In some sports, beta-blockers are used as performance-enhancing drugs. Beta-blockers are thought to have a favorable effect in shooting sports, because the decreased HR is less disturbing when aiming, and because the drugs suppress shaking of the hands.

Jet Lag

When the athlete travels through time zones, the day and night rhythm is disturbed. Most processes within the body are influenced by this day and night rhythm, and disturbance of this rhythm may harm performance capacity for some days. Traveling to the west can be tolerated more easily than traveling eastward. Athletes are advised to take 1 day of acclimatization per hour of time difference. So for a time difference of 7 hours, the athlete would need an adaptation period of 1 week. In the period before the trip, the athlete could get a head start on this adaptation by going to sleep extra early or extra late.

After arrival, the athlete should immediately take on the day and night rhythm of the new surroundings. Short naps in between delay the adaptation. Training should be adjusted temporarily. Continuing normal training activities despite the greater fatigue may result in overtraining. The athlete can check how she or he is adapting by measuring the HR. In the acclimatization period, both HRrest and the HR during exercise are higher. When HR returns to normal levels, the adaptation is complete and the athlete can train normally again.

Infectious Disease

Most athletes will encounter acute infectious diseases during their sports career. These diseases are a widespread problem, and in the world of sports they are often handled the wrong way. Athletes often continue their normal training because they underestimate the importance of the symptoms or because they worry about falling behind in training because of rest and inactivity. Those who work with athletes—the coaches, the sponsors, and the medical staff—generally would like to see the athletes continue training instead of taking the necessary rest. Unfortunately, many athletes lose a complete season because they did not let a simple flu run its course.

An infection may be disastrous for an athlete. Many people in other professions can continue working even with a bad cold, but top athletic achievement under these conditions is impossible. Even a light cold will decrease performance capacity by some 20%. Thus, athletes are well advised to take more rest and to diminish training drastically during infectious diseases. Only then will the body have a chance of recovering properly.

When fever is present, sports activities are absolutely prohibited. With every degree of temperature increase, HR increases by 10 to 15 bpm. Also during recovery from an infectious disease, HRrest is higher. And in the presence of fever, HR during submaximal effort shows a different pattern. Therefore, it is advisable to make some HR curves when the athlete is in good health and good condition. Make these HR measurements under equal circumstances. A cyclist may choose an ergometer, and for a runner a treadmill would be ideal; thus, the external conditions, such as temperature and front wind, are constant. For example, the athlete can make three standard measurements of 10 minutes at HRs of 130, 140, and 150, noting the distance reached and the pace.

During infectious diseases, HR measurements will show that performance capacity has diminished. Whenever performance is distinctly less than the normal level, the infection has not yet gone completely and the training program should be adjusted accordingly. When the HR curves have gone back to normal and the athlete feels better, training may resume. The workloads should be increased gradually to avoid overtraining, injuries, and disappointment.

When beginning training after an infectious disease, the athlete should train only at the level of a recovery workout or light endurance training. When things go well, as indicated by the HR measurements that were made under equal circumstances, the duration and intensity of training can be increased gradually. Graph 38 compares HRs in the absence and presence of infectious disease.

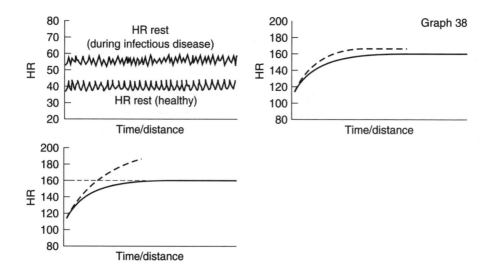

Mental Exercise

Another factor that can influence HR is mental stress. It is a recognized fact that difficult mental jobs can be very taxing. When such a job must be done in noisy surroundings or after a sleepless night, the effect on the body is even worse. The burden of mental jobs can be measured accurately by measuring the variations in HR. The average HR is about 60 bpm, that is, about one beat per second, with some minor variations. Mental activity seems to influence these variations. It appears that there is more variation (i.e., the HR is less regular) during times of mental stress.

Environmental Temperature

The curve in graph 39 (page 52) is for a half marathon run by a 43-year-old marathon runner with an HRdefl of 175. During the first 40 minutes of the half marathon, during which the weather is dry and the temperature is 16 degrees Celsius (61 degrees Fahrenheit), the runner's performance is excellent. This part of the race is run just below the HRdefl. In the 35th minute of the race, it starts to rain torrentially and the temperature drops. The runner cools enormously, cannot maintain his HR at the same high level, and experiences a loss in running pace.

Graph 40 shows the effect of a varying ambient temperature on a rower at rest. High temperature and humidity cause the elevation of HR in a sauna bather (curve shown in graph 41.)

Humidity and Body Temperature

For all exercise, whatever the volume or intensity, there is an optimal surrounding temperature and air humidity.

All physical actions depend on intricate chemical reactions in muscles and nerves. These reactions are very sensitive to variations in temperature, so changes in the internal body temperature affect performance. Although the body has a mechanism to regulate heat, internal body temperature may be affected by muscular activity or a high or low external temperature.

When body temperature is higher, physical processes run faster; in lower temperatures, they are slower. HR shows the lowest value at an outside temperature of about 20 degrees Celsius (68 degrees Fahrenheit). At rest, the body produces about 4.2 kilojoules (1 kilocalorie) per kilogram of body weight per hour. During physical exercise, the heat production of the body may rise to 42 to 84 kilojoules (10 to 20 kilocalories) per kilogram per hour. Therefore, great demands are placed on the body's heat regulation system. HR will increase, resulting in a better blood flow in the capillaries in the skin and increased production of perspiration. Equal exercise intensity with a body temperature of either 37 or 38 degrees Celsius (99 or 100 degrees Fahrenheit) shows a difference in HR by 10 to 15 bpm.

With a body temperature of 41 degrees Celsius (106 degrees Fahrenheit) or more, a so-called heatstroke may occur. Important factors for the occurrence

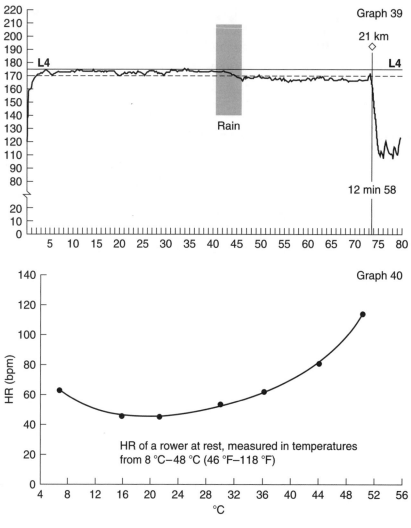

Graph 39

21 km

L4   L4

Rain

12 min 58

Graph 40

HR of a rower at rest, measured in temperatures
from 8 °C–48 °C (46 °F–118 °F)

°C

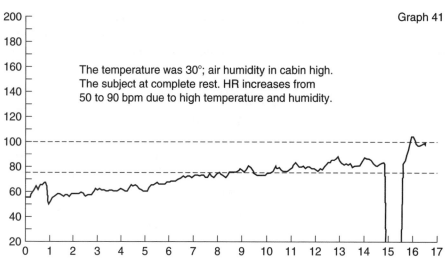

Graph 41

The temperature was 30°; air humidity in cabin high.
The subject at complete rest. HR increases from
50 to 90 bpm due to high temperature and humidity.

of a heatstroke during physical exercise are a high surrounding temperature, high air humidity, insufficient ventilation of the body, and insufficient fluid intake before the effort. It is of major importance to compensate for fluid loss by drinking 100 to 200 milliliters with short intervals. Fluid loss may be estimated by weighing the body regularly before and after workouts or races. During an endurance effort in the heat, a fluid loss of 1% to 3% of the body weight may occur after 1 to 2 hours. For an athlete weighing 70 kilograms, this means a fluid loss of 2.1 kilograms. This fluid loss decreases the circulating blood volume and diminishes the blood supply to the heart, which the body compensates for by increasing HR.

High surrounding temperature and a high degree of air humidity place greater demands on the human body during physical exercise. If the workload remains equal with an increasing surrounding temperature and/or air humidity, HR will increase. Performance capacity decreases to the same degree as temperature and air humidity increase. The enormous amount of heat released by muscular activity leads to a high internal body temperature despite increased heat regulation. This temperature increases even more when the workload becomes more intensive and longer and when external temperature and air humidity rise. In such situations, body temperature may increase up to 42 degrees Celsius (108 degrees Fahrenheit). This high body temperature is a distinctly limiting factor. In general, temperatures up to 20 degrees Celsius (68 degrees Fahrenheit) are favorable for endurance sports. Higher temperatures, between 25 and 35 degrees Celsius (77 and 95 degrees Fahrenheit), are favorable when fast power is required, as for sprints, throwing, and jumping.

Acclimatization to Heat

Athletes who want to participate in events in the tropics should be aware that the high temperatures in these areas are accompanied by a high degree of air humidity. A period of acclimatization to the heat is essential. When the athlete performs sports in a surrounding temperature of 36 degrees Celsius (97 degrees Fahrenheit), the body cannot get rid of its own heat production. In addition, a high air humidity limits the evaporation of sweat, which limits the cooling that can take place due to evaporation. On account of this minimal heat release, body temperature will rise.

After a period of acclimatization, the body starts perspiring sooner, even at a lower body temperature. This enhances cooling, and sweat production increases. Under normal conditions the perspiration glands can produce 1.8 liters of sweat per hour. Through acclimatization, sweat production may practically double to 3.5 liters per hour. Maximum sweat production may be as high as 10 liters per day. Tour de France riders may have a fluid intake from 10 to 15 liters per 24 hours during warmer days. After acclimatization, the salt content of sweat diminishes and the salt balance is disturbed less quickly. The eventual result is that after acclimatization, the body can cope with heat more effectively. But an

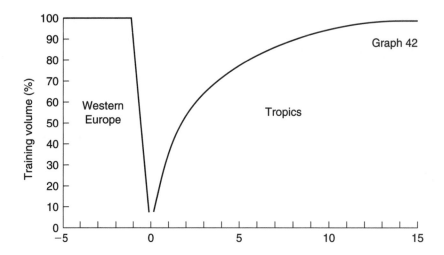

adequate fluid intake remains essential, because the beneficial effects of acclimatization diminish rapidly in case of dehydration (fluid loss). A period of 3 to 4 weeks seems ideal for a good acclimatization, but at least 10 days is essential. The best location for acclimatization is, of course, the place where the race will be. The athlete who takes ample time to get used to the heat will compensate for the loss of performance capacity that occurs in the first few days. In the beginning a normal training program will not be possible because of the heat. Graph 42 shows how training levels are affected by heat and humidity.

The opposite is also true: People who live constantly in air-conditioned surroundings may lose their capacity for perspiration, because their sweat glands become inactive. When they go outside on a hot day, they are at risk for a heatstroke.

It is not absolutely necessary to sleep or rest in hot surroundings, but if a good night's sleep is not affected by heat there is no objection to it. If, on the other hand, the athlete sleeps poorly because of the heat, it is advisable to rest in an air-conditioned room. A good night's sleep remains very important.

Those who cannot afford to acclimatize for 3 to 4 weeks can start working on heat adaptation at home. This is possible by spending about 90 to 120 minutes per day in climate rooms or well-regulated saunas. The advantage is that this method leaves ample time for normal training activities. The effects of acclimatization disappear after 4 to 8 weeks of nonexposure to heat.

Finally, in high temperatures, the warm-up period should be shorter than normal and preferably should be in the shade or in a cool room. Diminishing heat production within the body before the race might enhance performance.

Heat Problems

Heatstroke is a major heat-related problem for athletes. In 85% of heatstrokes that occur due to an athletic event, a collapse takes place after the finish, and only 15% collapse during the race. Athletes who have a normal coordination who collapse after the finish go through a vasovagal collapse, because stopping muscular activity can cause a considerable and abrupt drop in blood pressure. The rectal temperature of these athletes will not be higher than 40 degrees Celsius (104 degrees Fahrenheit). An athlete who has collapsed from heat should be placed in a horizontal position with the legs elevated to readjust the oxygen flow to the brain. This simple action is often enough to reverse the collapse. A collapse before the finish is often a heatstroke, in which case immediate cooling is essential. The athlete should not attempt to finish.

The number of heat collapses increases with the level of training. Elite athletes can cope with the highest level of activity and therefore reach the highest body temperature. The largest number of heat collapses takes place during short intensive races in hot and humid surroundings.

Symptoms of Heat Problems

- Rectal temperature of 40 degrees Celsius (104 degrees Fahrenheit) or higher
- Athlete often feels cool because of diminished superficial blood flow
- "Goose pimples," headache, tingling arms, "hot" head
- Often diminished sweat production

An athlete becomes thirsty after loss of only 1% of his/her body weight. The feeling of thirst often defines the onset of dehydration. If the athlete is really dehydrated, fluid loss should be compensated for, which can only be done by infusion.

To treat a heatstroke, immediately remove the athlete from the heat (sun) and start cooling immediately. Submerging the athlete in ice water helps to decrease temperature rapidly. If submersion is not possible, put as many ice packs as possible on the athlete's body, especially the armpits, the neck, and groin, or put the athlete under a cold shower. To avoid hypothermia, stop cooling when the temperature drops below 39 degrees Celsius (102 degrees Fahrenheit). Check the athlete's temperature every 15 minutes for the next hour.

Important Advice
for Physical Exercise in Tropical Conditions

- Start acclimatizing long before the race.
- Start training in hot weather.
- Track dehydration by weighing the body and checking urine for frequency, color, and quantity.
- Avoid alcohol and caffeine.

- Use only those beverages the athlete is used to, with sufficient carbohydrates and electrolytes. The drink should be hypotonous.

- Compensate for salt and fluid loss via meals.

- Get a good night's sleep, even if this means sleeping in an air-conditioned room or with a fan.

- Limit the duration of the warm-up to minimize the increase in body temperature.

- Warm up in the shade or in a cool room.

- Adjust drinking habits to the heat. Choose a good sports drink, and drink even if not thirsty.

- To diagnose heatstroke, always take temperature rectally. In case of collapse, consider other causes.

HR Curves of Acclimatization to Tropical Surroundings

Basic Details

Experienced marathon runner

Recent HRdefl: 174

Recovery runs: HR 140 to 145 (about 13 kilometers per hour)

Endurance runs: HR 150 to 160 (about 14.5 kilometers per hour)

Intensive workouts: HR 160 to 170 (about 16 kilometers per hour)

Tolerance: HR 170 to 180 (about 17.5 kilometers per hour)

HRmax: 185

Target

Marathon race in the tropics with an adaptation period of 12 days. Equatorial area in the wet monsoon period: no direct sun, high air humidity of about 95%. Minimum nighttime temperature 24 degrees Celsius (75 degrees Fahrenheit), in daytime 30 to 37 degrees Celsius (86 to 99 degrees Fahrenheit).

First measurement after 3 days of getting used to the climate and time change via short jogs (see graph 43).

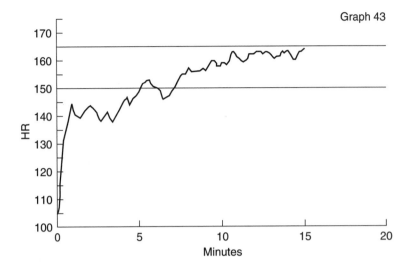

Graph 43

<table>
<tr><td></td></tr>
</table>

HR / Minutes

DAY 3 Fifteen-minute workout at jogging pace (about 12 kilometers per hour); equal level of exercise. Subjective feeling of heaviness from the 5th minute. Until 5 minutes, values are normal. After that, there is a striking increase of HR from 150 to 160; after 10 minutes, there is another increase to 165. So the exercise seems to be too heavy even with a minimal pace (see graph 44).

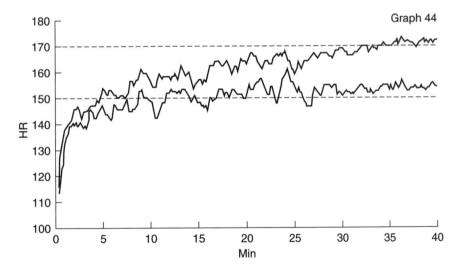

Graph 44

HR / Min

DAY 4

Early morning. Forty-minute workout at low to normal training pace (13 to 14 kilometers per hour) Again, HR is far above normal in comparison with pace. HR cannot be stabilized. After 30 minutes HR increases to 170, the limit for tolerance.

DAY 5

Evening. Identical workout as previous day. This is the beginning of adaptation, and there is distinct improvement. With an equal load and lower HR, the HR curve begins to flatten (see graph 45).

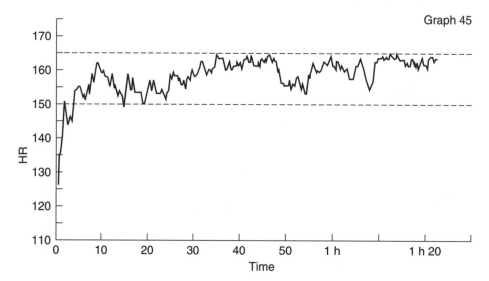

Graph 45

DAY 6

First longer workout is possible. One hour and 20 minutes at normal endurance pace (13 to 14 kilometers per hour). HR is still rather high for this type of exercise, range 155 to 165, but is reasonably flat (see graph 46).

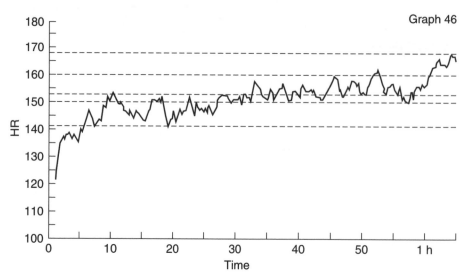

Graph 46

DAY 7 Longer endurance run: 1 hour and 5 minutes (13 to 14 kilometers per hour). HR is still too high (see graph 47).

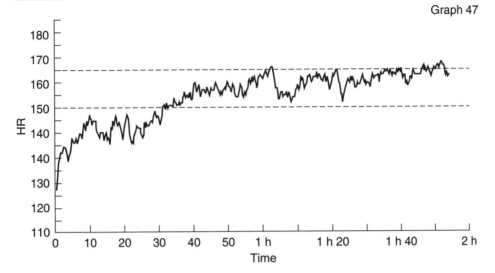

Graph 47

DAY 8 First extra-long endurance run: 25 kilometers in 1 hour and 55 minutes (about 13 kilometers per hour). HR still tends to gradually increase. Despite a decrease in the pace to normal values of 12 to 13 kilometers per hour, the HR keeps increasing to tolerance level. The progress of adaptation can be seen in the duration of exercise that can be handled: 2 hours, compared with 15 minutes in the first days (see graph 48).

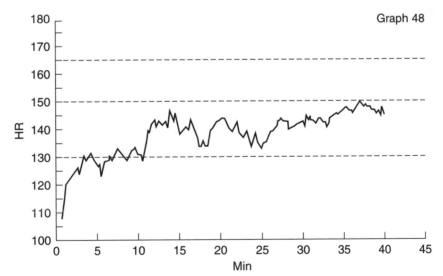

Graph 48

DAY 9 Forty-minute workout (13 to 14 kilometers per hour). Acclimatization seems complete. Despite the effort, subjectively felt very heavy. HR does not go much higher than 150 (see graph 49).

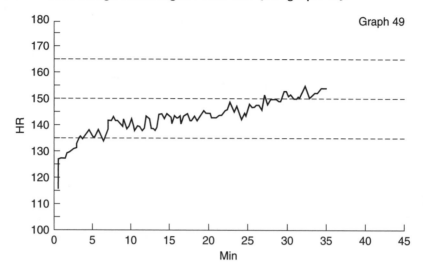

Graph 49

DAY 10 Thirty-five-minute endurance run (13 to 14 kilometers per hour). Despite the heaviness of the effort, HR is under control. Acclimatization may be considered complete.

DAY 11 Day of rest before the marathon. Based on HR measurements from 11 days of adaptation, related to the pace and the very high effort, the HR in the race should not surpass 160, which means that the pace will not be more than 4 minutes per kilometer.

DAY 12 Marathon starts at 6.00 A.M. Expected speed is 15 kilometers per hour. Temperature 26 degrees Celsius (79 degrees Fahrenheit). After sunrise, temperature expected to increase to 35 degrees Celsius (95 degrees Fahrenheit) (see graph 50).

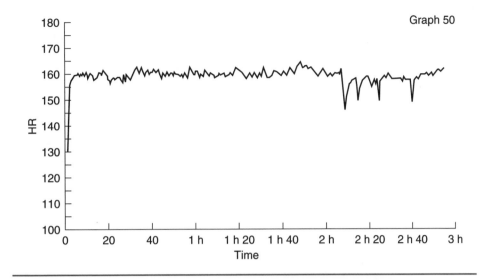

Strikingly stable and flat HR that can practically be kept up to the finish: Analysis of the adaptation and prediction of the performance seem correct. In Europe, the same HR would yield a time of 2.40. Moreover, a higher HR (e.g., 170) would have been possible in Europe, which would have meant a time of about 2.25 or 2.30. Marathon times in the tropics are 15 to 25 minutes more, according to the experiences of European runners. A time loss of 10 to 15 minutes seems minimal (see graph 51).

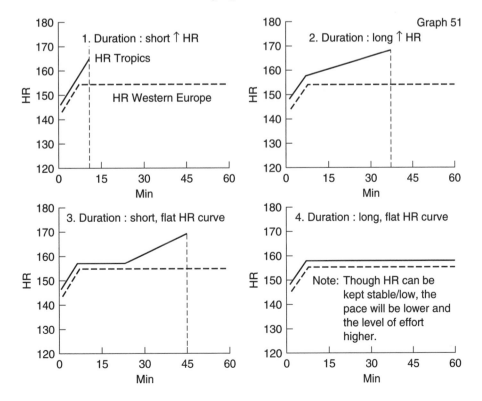

During physical exercise, much heat is produced. Perspiration is an important means of heat release, but a high fluid loss can cause serious complications. Body temperature during physical exercise may increase to 40 to 41 degrees Celsius (104 to 106 degrees Fahrenheit). Body weight may decrease by many kilograms due to fluid loss. Whenever fluid loss is more than 3% of the body weight, the internal body temperature will rise and a life-threatening situation may occur.

The curve in graph 52 reflects the course of the HR during endurance load at 70% of the maximum oxygen consumption. The temperature during the test was 20 degrees Celsius (68 degrees Fahrenheit). The test was ended when the runner was exhausted. No fluid intake during the test caused a higher HR, and exhaustion was reached half an hour sooner. Drinking 250 milliliters every 15 minutes kept the HR at a constant level. The duration in the fluid intake test was considerably longer.

Fluid loss, which is disadvantageous to performance capacity, can be compensated for by drinking regularly. Also, repeated cooling during exercise in hot surroundings may slow fluid loss, reducing the decrease in performance (see graph 53).

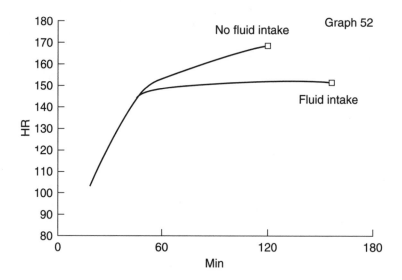

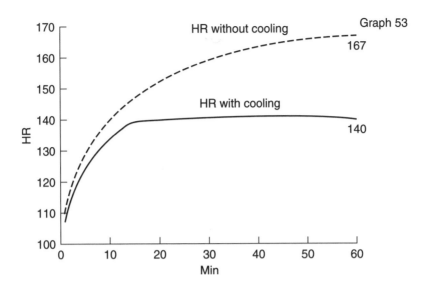

The positive effects of cooling during exercise are clear. In one experiment, an athlete was tested two times on a bicycle ergometer with 4 days between tests. The first test took place without cooling, but during the second test, the body was kept wet with wet sponges and a fan. Other conditions in both tests were identical. The temperature was 25 degrees Celsius (77 degrees Fahrenheit), and relative humidity was constant. Total duration of the cycling test was 60 minutes. In the test without cooling, HR gradually increased from 135 to 167 bpm. In the test with cooling, HR settled at a constant level of 140 bpm. Thus, cooling may enable the athlete to maintain exercise longer.

Cycling is faster than running, so cooling by means of air is greater during cycling. The more moderate running pace provides less air cooling and increases fluid loss, with all its unfavorable consequences. Cooling too fast with water that is too cold can be detrimental. The superficial blood vessels then cramp, and superfluous heat cannot be released. The best way to avoid premature exhaustion during exercise in hot conditions is to drink regularly and wet the body with a sponge periodically.

chapter 3

The Deflection Point

The Italian physiology professor Francesco Conconi developed a noninvasive method of determining the deflection point without measuring lactate and thus without taking blood samples. The deflection point (HRdefl) may be defined as the heart rate (HR) above which lactate accumulation will increase. As a rule, lactate content at the HRdefl is about 4 millimoles per liter. Exercise at the level of the HRdefl may be maintained for a long period of time, because there is an equilibrium in the production and elimination of lactate. From Conconi's publication (Conconi et al. 1982), it appears that there is a good correlation between the anaerobic threshold and the HRdefl.

The anaerobic threshold means that above this level of exercise, lactate content will greatly increase. Lactate content at the anaerobic threshold is also about 4 millimoles per liter. This chapter will discuss Conconi's test as well as the Åstrand test, the maximal test, and the individual anaerobic threshold (IAT).

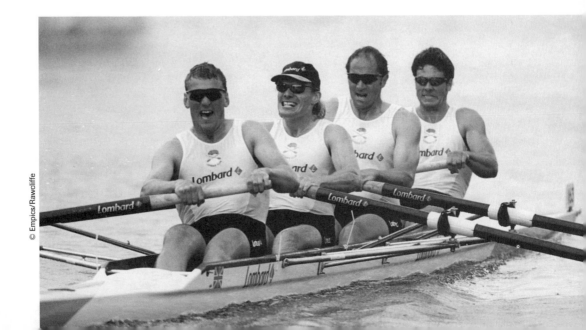

© Empics/Rawcliffe

Conconi's Test

Conconi's test is carried out as follows (Conconi used well-trained athletes for his tests): In a field test, the HR and the running pace are taken according to a certain protocol. An extensive warm-up of 15 to 30 minutes is followed by an uninterrupted endurance run. During this run the pace is quickened slightly at regular intervals, not more than half a kilometer per hour. After this acceleration the pace is kept at a constant level again. HR is registered every last 50 meters. Because time is also registered, the pace can be calculated. The maximum pace eventually reached varies from 18 to 25 kilometers per hour depending on the condition of the athlete. The relation between HR and running pace is partially linear and partially nonlinear. The pace at which the linear relation is lost is the HRdefl. The time that the HR needs to adapt to the new pace is 10 to 20 seconds. This only applies when the increase in running pace is not more than half a kilometer per hour.

The nonlinear part of the curve comparing running pace and HR can best be measured with a protocol in which running pace is accelerated every 200 meters. With this protocol, the number of measuring points above the HRdefl is greatest so that the best curve can be constructed.

This curve in graph 54 runs linearly up to HR 190 and a running pace of 21.1 kilometers per hour. At higher speeds there is a deflection in the curve. For this athlete, the HRdefl is 190. His pace at the deflection, also called the V4 pace, is 21.1 kilometers per hour. The letter V stands for velocity, so V4 is the pace at the HRdefl: the pace corresponding to a blood lactate of 4 millimoles per liter.

The left curve in graph 55 reflects the relationship between pace and HR. The right curve reflects the relationship between pace and lactate. The bend in the HR curve is the HRdefl, which corresponds to a certain pace. The bend in the lactate curve is the anaerobic threshold. The graph shows that the

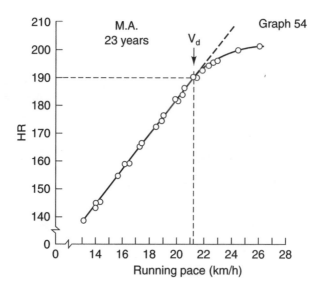

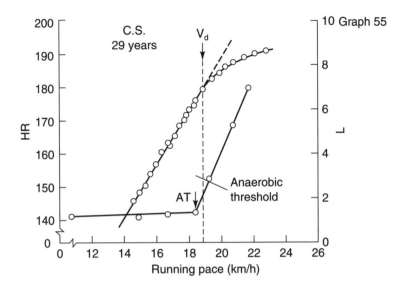

HRdefl and the anaerobic threshold can be found at nearly the same pace. In well-trained athletes, HRdefl is 5 to 20 (average 10.6) beats per minute (bpm) lower than maximum HR (HRmax). In untrained persons, the HR at the deflection point is 20 to 27 bpm lower than HRmax. When the field test is repeated with the same person a few days later, the same results will be obtained. So Conconi's test can be reproduced well.

Graph 56 demonstrates the shift in the running pace–HR curve. After a training period, the curve shifts for both runners. Whenever condition is improved, the curve moves to the right. The third test on May 30, with S.A., was done some days before the athlete was diagnosed with mononucleosis. The curve already shows a decrease in performance capacity. The Conconi curve will reflect overtraining, infections, or any change in condition.

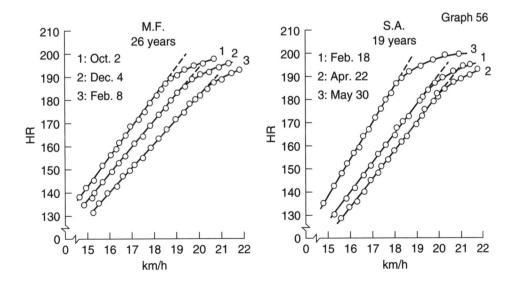

The linear relationship between pace and HR is lost at high running paces. There is a good correlation between the deflection pulse (Dp) and the anaerobic threshold. When the pace is accelerated to a point above the Dp or anaerobic threshold, lactate will accumulate rapidly. This accumulation of lactate is a signal that aerobic energy supply is lagging behind. Anaerobic energy supply comes into play as a kind of emergency system.

There is a fixed relationship between running pace and the pace of a 5,000-meter race, a marathon, and a 1-hour time trial. During the 1-hour run, the pace is practically the same as the V4 pace. During the 5,000-meter, the anaerobic system is constantly called on so that running pace may reach a point above the V4 pace. The share of the anaerobic system in energy supply during a 5,000-meter race is about 10%. In a marathon, the pace is distinctly below the V4 pace. Investigations indicate that the pace of the marathon is about 95% of the V4 pace.

Practical Application of Conconi's Test for Runners

The athlete starts with a 15- to 20-minute warm-up. Then the actual test begins on a 400-meter track. The pace at the onset of the test is low and depends on the athlete's condition. Untrained persons run the first 200 meters in about 70 seconds, and well-trained athletes in 60 seconds. After every 200 meters, the pace is accelerated, so that every consecutive 200 meters is run about 2 seconds faster. At the end of every 200 meters, the HR and pace are recorded. The athlete continues to increase the pace after every 200 meters and keeps the new pace constant. The test continues until the athlete cannot accelerate any more (see graph 57).

Figure 3.1 shows that the test begins with both the runner and a helper at Point 1. At Point 2, the athlete registers his or her HR and accelerates immediately for the next 200 meters. After returning to Point 1, the athlete again registers his or her HR and shouts to the helper what the HR values were at the

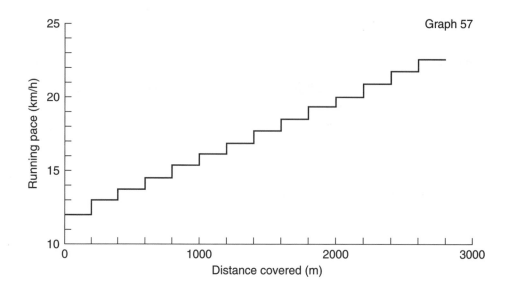

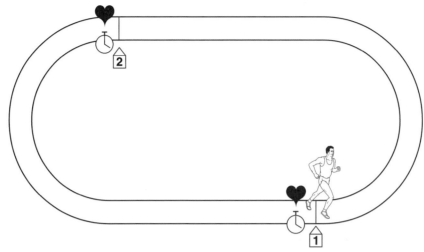

Figure 3.1 Test method on 400-meter track.

first 200-meter segment and the second 200 meter segment. So at Point 1, the times and HRs for each 200-meter segment are always recorded. With this protocol, the number of recordings is 12 to 16. Total running time will be between 10 and 12 minutes with a total distance between 2,400 and 3,200 meters.

Requirements for the Test

HR monitor

Stopwatch

The protocol charts

Pen or pencil

400-meter track

Lap time = time per 200 meters

Figure 3.2 shows the pace in kilometers per hour. For example, if the 200-meter lap time is 50 seconds, the pace is 14.4 kilometers per hour. The minutes per kilometer bar on the right side of figure 3.2 gives the time per kilometer that corresponds to that pace. The athlete or coach should plot the data on 1-millimeter graph paper, where the vertical or y-axis represents the HR and the horizontal or x-axis represents pace in kilometers per hour. As shown in graph 58, HR values are plotted with the running pace.

When all the dots are put in place, the curve is drawn. The bend in the curve, which corresponds to Dp, is usually around an HR of 210 minus age. After drawing this curve, the athlete knows what pace or HR corresponds to the anaerobic threshold. Thus, Conconi's test provides information about the condition of the athlete (see table 3.1). Training advice may be based on the tests, and the impact of a training period can be established.

Time 200m	km/h	Time 1000m
sec. 70	10	6' 00"
65	11	5' 30"
60	12	5' 00"
55	13	4' 30"
50	14	
	15	4 00"
45	16	
	17	3' 30"
40	18	
39	19	
38		
37		
36	20	3'00"
35	21	
34		
33	22	
32		
31	23	
30	24	2' 30"
29	25	
28	26	
27		
	27	
26	28	
25	29	
24	30	2' 00"

Count	Road	♥	⏱	km/h
1	200			
2	400			
3	600			
4	800			
5	1000			
6	1200			
7	1400			
8	1600			
9	1800			
10	2000			
11	2200			
12	2400			
13	2600			
14	2800			
15	3000			
16	3200			
17	3400			
18	3600			

Figure 3.2 Test data.

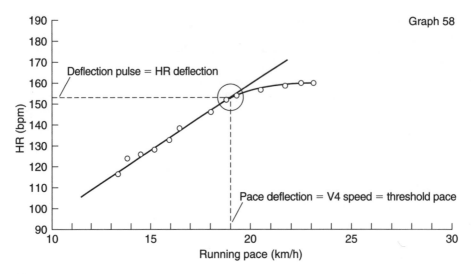

Table 3.1 Athlete's Condition

Condition	V4 (km/h)
Very bad	9.0
Bad	10.0
Sufficient	12.0
Excellent	14.0
Swiss marathon champion	19.0
World record marathon	23.6

Graph 59 (page 72) shows the distinction between endurance workouts in the aerobic area and intervals in the anaerobic area. The V4 pace is 100%.

The various training intensities may be deduced from the V4 pace (see table 3.2).

After 1 month of training, the test can be repeated under the same circumstances. If endurance capacity has improved, the curve shifts to the right, as in graph 60. If endurance capacity has deteriorated, the curve shifts to the left. Conconi's test is useful only when the athlete has rested well enough and is in reasonable condition. The athlete must be able to handle a 45-minute endurance run.

In practice, it takes much experience to have such a feeling for pace that every 200-meter segment can be run 2 seconds faster. Therefore, Conconi's test is made easier with the help of a prerecorded cassette tape.

Table 3.2 Training Advice

Endurance runs		
Pace	**Intensity (%)**	**Duration (min)**
Slow	75	90-120
Quiet	80	50-90
Intermediate	90	30-50
Fast	97	20-30
Intervals		
Long	100	6-12
Short	103	3-6

Note: The V4 pace is 100%.

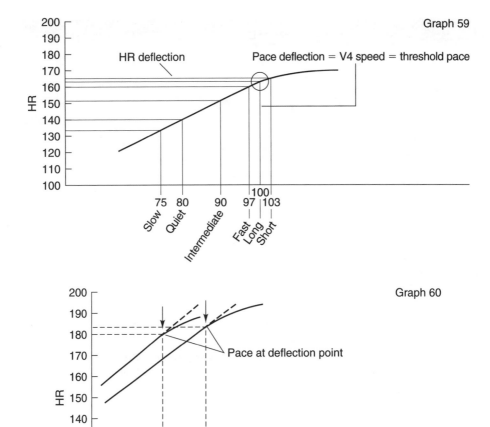

Requirements for administering Conconi's test using a cassette tape

- Athletics track with a visible mark every 20 meters
- Table with calculated times when every 20-meter mark should be passed
- Light, portable tape player with headphones
- Pouch with a clip to fasten the tape player
- Cassette tape with prerecorded signals when marks should be passed (to be recorded with a simple cassette recorder)
- HR monitor with memory function
- Table for calculating and plotting the data after the test (see table 3.3).

Table 3.3 Recorded Signal Times

Mark distance	Time (min/sec)	Mark distance	Time (min/sec)	Mark distance	Time (min/sec)	Mark distance	Time (min/sec)
2	00:06	2	3:47.5	2	6:48.4	2	9:18.4
4	00:12	4	3:52.4	4	6:52.4	4	9:21.8
6	00:18	6	3:57.3	6	6.56.5	6	9:25.2
8	00:24	8	4:02.2	8	7:00.5	8	9:28.6
10	00:30	10	4:07.1	10	7:04.5	10	9:32.0
2	00:36	2	4:11.9	2	7:08.5	2	9:35.3
4	00:42	4	4:16.8	4	7:12.5	4	9:38.7
6	00:48	6	4:21.7	6	7:16.6	6	9:42.1
8	00:54	8	4:26.6	8	7:20.6	8	9:45.5
10	00:60	10	4:31.5	10	7:24.6	10	9:48.9
2	1:05.7	2	4:36.2	2	7:28.4	2	9:52.2
4	1:11.4	4	4:40.8	4	7:32.3	4	9:55.4
6	1:22.8	6	4:45.5	6	7:36.1	6	9:58.7
8	1:17.1	8	4:50.1	8	7:40.0	8	10.02.0
10	1:28.5	10	4:54.8	10	7:43.8	10	10.05.3
2	1:34.2	2	4:59.4	2	7:47.6	2	10.06.5
4	1:39.9	4	5:04.1	4	7:51.5	4	10:11.8
6	1:45.6	6	5:06.7	6	7:55.3	6	10:15.1
8	1:51.3	8	5:13.4	8	7:59.2	8	10:18.3
400	1:57.0	1,200	5:18.0	2,000	8:03.0	2,800	10:21.6
2	2:02.4	2	5:22.4	2	8:06.7	2	10:24.8
4	2:07.8	4	5:26.9	4	8:10.4	4	10:27.9
6	2:13.2	6	5:31.3	6	8:14.0	6	10:31.1
8	2:18.7	8	5:35.7	8	8:17.7	8	10:34.3
10	2:24.1	10	5:40.1	10	8:21.4	10	10:37.4
2	2:29.5	2	5:44.6	2	8:25.1	2	10:40.6
4	2:34.9	4	5:49.0	4	8:28.7	4	10:43.8
6	2:40.3	6	5:53.4	6	8:32.4	6	10:46.9
8	2:45.7	8	5:57.8	8	8:36.1	8	10:50.1
10	2:51.2	10	6:02.3	10	8:39.8	10	10:53.3
2	2:56.3	2	6:06.5	2	8:43.3	2	10:56.3
4	3:01.4	4	6:10.7	4	8:46.8	4	10:59.4
6	3:06.6	6	6:14.9	6	8:50.3	6	11:02.5
8	3:11.7	8	6:19.1	8	8:53.9	8	11:05.6
10	3:16.9	10	6:23.3	10	8:57.4	10	11:08.6
2	3:22.0	2	6:27.5	2	9:00.9	2	11:11.7
4	3:27.2	4	6:31.8	4	9:04.4	4	11:14.8
6	3:32.3	6	6:35.0	6	9.08.0	6	11:17.9
8	3:37.5	8	6:40.2	8	9:11.5	8	11:20.9
800	3:42.6	1,600	6.44.4	2,400	9:15.0	3,200	11.24.0

Note: At the beginning of the test every 200-m step is run 2-3 sec faster. Later on in the test every next 200-m step is run 1-2 sec faster.

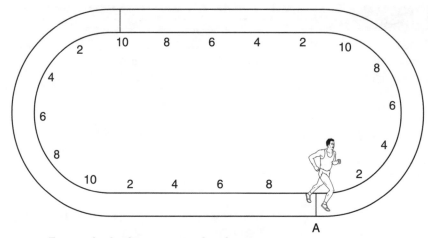

Figure 3.3 Test method using cassette signals.

Before beginning the test, the athlete should ensure that the tape player and HR monitor are functioning correctly. It is advisable to wear the HR monitor during the warm-up. The athlete starts with a warm-up of 15 to 20 minutes. Then the actual test begins on a 400-meter track. The starting pace is low but is accelerated every 200 meters. Every subsequent 200-meter segment is run about 2 seconds faster.

The athlete, equipped with a portable tape player and HR monitor, starts at Point A, as shown in figure 3.3. The athlete runs at a pace that is dictated via the headphones, until he or she cannot reach the marks on time any more.

The test series starts with a warm-up of 2 minutes in which the workload rises to 200 or 250 watts, depending on the athlete's condition. Then the athlete pedals at 200 or 250 watts during 6 minutes. With the HR reached after 6 minutes, the $\dot{V}O_2$max can be estimated with the help of some tables; then the condition figure can be calculated. This is the well-known Åstrand test.

Åstrand Test

The Åstrand test is also used to determine an athlete's condition. This test measures the athlete's condition by means of a linear relationship between HR and the level of exercise. In an Åstrand test, condition is determined by counting HR during one submaximal effort. It is a fast and easy method of determining maximal oxygen consumption ($\dot{V}O_2$max). The higher the $\dot{V}O_2$max (expressed in liters per minute), the better the athlete's condition.

For this test we use a Monark ergometer with a mechanical brake. After a 3-minute warm-up, one constant submaximal effort is made during 6 minutes. Try to choose a workload that elicits HR values somewhere between 140 and 160 bpm. Pedaling frequency is 50 revolutions per minute (RPM). By the end of the test, HR will have settled at one constant level.

A 25-year-old athlete with a body weight of 70 kilograms cycles at a constant load of 200 watts. After 6 minutes his heart rate is 146 bpm. His $\dot{V}O_2$max is 4.8 liters per minute. To determine his condition figure, the $\dot{V}O_2$max in milliliters is divided by body weight in kilograms; thus, $4.8 \times 1{,}000$ milliliters per minute $\div 70 = 68.6$ milliliters per kilogram per minute.

Body weight plays an important role in many endurance sports (heavy athletes with a high $\dot{V}O_2$max have a lower conditioning level because of their body weight). The $\dot{V}O_2$max and the conditioning level are important values for an endurance athlete. By regularly undergoing an Åstrand test, the athlete can keep good tabs on his or her condition.

After the Åstrand test, the athlete undergoes a 2-minute cool-down at 75 watts. After that the maximal test begins. When the test person cannot continue, the test is ended. Refer to graphs 62-64.

Maximal Test

A third test is the maximal test. In this test, a constant total workload is maintained per segment, but the segments decrease in time as the test continues. In our protocol the first segment is 90 seconds, and the last is only 32 seconds. HR is measured continually during the test, and the HR at which the athlete starts gasping is recorded. Other measurements include body weight, body length, skinfolds to calculate fat percentage, and blood pressure before and after the effort. The test is performed on a Lode ergometer with a constant pedaling frequency of 90 RPM, which is checked conscientiously. The test ends when the athlete cannot keep up the desired effort, or when pedaling frequency can no longer be maintained.

Using the same principles, these tests can also be used for cyclists. The protocol and an example are illustrated here.

An example of testing and training advice is given for a top-performing cyclist Bart Brentjens. He did Conconi's test, the Åstrand test, the maximal test, and the anaerobic threshold test.

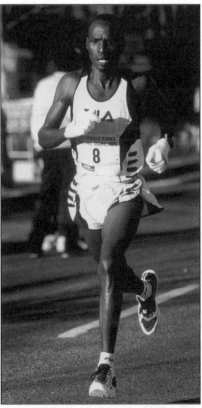

© Photo Run

Ultramarathoners, like Simon Bor, can use Conconi's test to determine HR & deflection.

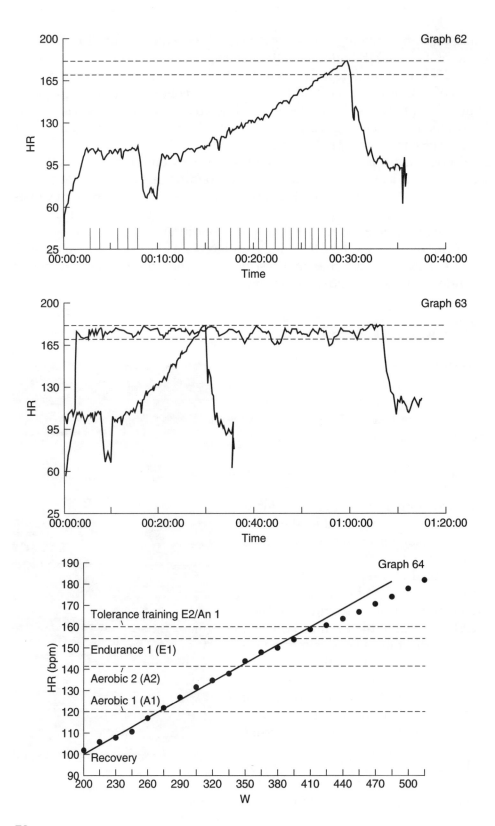

BART BRENTJENS

Sport: ATB

Category: pro

World Champion ATB 1995

Winner Tour de France/ATB 1995–1996

Dutch champion 1995

Olympic champion 1996

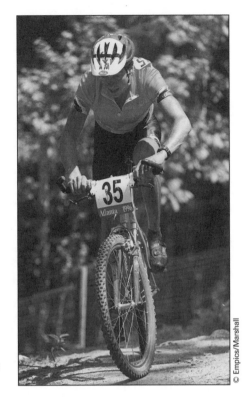

© Empics/Marshall

Bart Brentjens, Olympic champion ATB, 1996 Atlanta Games.

Training intensities

Recovery workouts: HR under 120
Aerobic workouts 1 (A1): HR between 120 and 142
Aerobic workouts 2 (A2): HR between 142 and 155
Endurance workouts 1 (E1): HR between 155 and 160
Endurance workouts 2 (E2): HR between 158 and 162
Anaerobic workouts 1 (An1): HR between 160 and HRmax

Test results

Name: Bart Brentjens

Birth: October 10, 1968

Test date: January 5, 1998

Time: 1:00 p.m.

Age: 27

Sex: male

Sport: ATB

Category: pro

Body length: 185 cm

Body weight: 78.4 kg

Sum of skinfolds: 24.8 mm

Fat percentage: 10.6%

Total fat mass: 8.3 kg

Fat-free mass: 70.1 kg

$\dot{V}O_2$**max:** 9.58 liters per minute

Condition figure: 122.19 milliliters per kilogram per minute

Blood pressure at rest: 120/70 mmHg

Blood pressure after test: 180/75 mmHg

HRrest: 36 bpm

HRdefl: 160 bpm

HRmax: 182 bpm

HR 1 minute after effort: 137 bpm at 75 watts 5% > average

HR 3 minutes after effort: 101 bpm at 75 watts 9% > average

HR 4 minutes after effort: 92 bpm at 75 watts 10% > average

Maximum power output: 515 watts

Maximum power output: 6.57 watts per kilogram of body weight

Power output at HRdefl: 455 watts

Power output at HRdefl: 5.80 watts per kilogram of body weight

Training advice

1. Warm-up
   a. 1 minute of pedal contact at 42 × 19
   b. 2 minutes at 42 × 21; 90 to 110 RPM
   c. 2 minutes at 42 × 19; 90 to 110 RPM
   d. Recovery: three to five rushes at 42 × 23 (5 seconds), and then three to five rushes 42 × 14 (5 seconds)

    e. 2 minutes at 42 × 19; 90 to 110 RPM

    f. 2 minutes at 42 × 17; 90 to 110 RPM

2. Recovery workout, RPM under 120

   Purpose: Remove by-products from muscles, acquire flexibility.

   Intensity: Not over A1 level

   This workout is done the day after a heavy race or workout, when the athlete has not quite recovered, and the day before a race.

3. Extensive aerobic workout (A1; HR 120 to 140)

   Purpose: Improve basic condition and endurance capacity.

   Aerobic workouts at low intensities improve

   - the capacity to burn fats;
   - aerobic energy supply, because the muscles can absorb and handle more oxygen; and
   - capillarization of the muscles.

   This workout involves extensive endurance training of long duration; intensity of recovery workouts should be 42 × 17 and less (16, 15, 14), 90 to 100 RPM.

4. Intensive aerobic workout (A2; HR 142 to 155) and extensive endurance workout (E1; HR 155 to 160)

   Purpose: Improve the speed that can be maintained for a long period of time without lactate accumulation.

   These workouts improve aerobic endurance capacity and the capacity to burn carbohydrates.

   A2 involves intensive aerobic training, 42 × 15 and smaller (15, 14, 13), 100 to 110 RPM, two to three blocks of 15 to 20 minutes, pause A1 for 3 to 10 minutes.

   E1 involves extensive endurance training, 42 × 19 and smaller (18, 17, 16), 110 RPM minimally, three to five blocks of 3 to 10 minutes, pause A1 for 3 to 10 minutes.

5. Intensive endurance workout (E2; HR 158 to 162) and anaerobic workout (An1; HR 160 to HRmax).

   Purpose: Increase speed in short, fierce power bursts (escapes, closing gaps); develop capacity to react to speed changes in races and possibility to repeat power bursts quickly.

Performing intervals and repetitions improves

- the capacity to tolerate high lactate content,
- the capacity to burn carbohydrates anaerobically, and
- the specific metabolism and coordination (feeling of cadence).

E2, duration of high-speed blocks that are long (52 × 17) and smaller (16, 15), lasting 3 to 10 minutes. Pause: equal to working interval, 3 to 10 minutes recovery, 42 × 17 (16).

An1, duration of high speed submaximal, 42 × 19 and smaller, minimally 110 RPM until legs get sore. Five to 20 blocks of 20 to 180 seconds. Pause 1 to 2 minutes, recovery.

An1, duration of high speed maximal, 42 × 19 and smaller (18, 17, 16), minimally 110 RPM until legs get sore. Five to 15 blocks of 40 to 50 seconds. Pause 3 minutes, recovery. Or, 3 to 10 blocks of 60 to 90 seconds. Pause 5 minutes, recovery.

6. Power training and cadence training Train especially those areas in which performance is poor. Do a good warm-up before training, and cool down for at least half an hour (recovery).

Fast power

52 × 14 (13) rushes, all-out sprints at maximum speed.

Pause: recovery, three to five series.

20 seconds, pause 3 minutes; 20 seconds, pause 3 minutes; 20 seconds, pause 3 minutes; 20 seconds, pause 6 minutes; and so on.

So this exercise involves 20 seconds of maximum effort with 3 minutes of recovery. Between the series, the athlete takes 6 minutes, of recovery.

Acceleration power

52 × 14/13 rushes, sprints starting from high speed (uphill or front wind 52 × 15/16). Five to 15 blocks at 5 to 10 seconds.

Pause 1 minute, recovery or 20 to 25 seconds.

Pause 3 minutes, recovery.

Endurance power submaximal

52 × 15 increasing intensity, intervals with decreasing pause.

Pause recovery, two to three times.

50 seconds, pause 7 minutes; 50 seconds, pause 5 minutes; 50 seconds, pause 3 minutes; 50 seconds, pause 1 minute; 50 seconds, pause 9 minutes; and so on.

Endurance power maximal

20 minutes of A1, then uphill or overpass or front wind.

3 × 10 at one or two cogs less on the sprocket wheel.

3 minutes all-out effort.

Pause 4 minutes, recovery.

Conconi's test for cyclists

Name:	Sport:
First name:	Category:
Address:	Date test:
Postal code:	Time:
Place:	
Age:	Date of birth:

Blood pressure at rest:	mmHg	Skinfolds		
Blood pressure after test:	mmHg	Biceps:	mm	
HR at rest:	bpm	Triceps:	mm	
HR gasping onset:	bpm	Subscapula:	mm	
HRmax:	bpm	Suprailiac:	mm	
HR 1 minute after test:	75 watts			
HR 5 minutes after test:	75 watts			
No. HR monitor:				
File number:				

Åstrand test

0-2 load rises linearly to 200 to 250 watts

3 min HR:

4 min HR:

5 min HR:

6 min HR:

7 min HR:

8 min HR:

Results of Åstrand test

$\dot{V}O_2$max: 1/min

Condition figure: ml/kg/min

Body weight: kg

Body length: cm

Fat percentage: %

Fat total: kg

Fat-free mass: kg

After 8 minutes, allow 2 minutes of rest (75 watts).

Table 3.4 can be used to record the HR of the cyclist being tested.

Table 3.4 Protocol for Conconi's Test for Cyclists

Cycling time (min:sec)	Duration of effort (sec)	Power (W)	HR (bpm)
11:30	90	200	
12:54	84	215	
14:12	78	230	
15:25	73	245	
16:34	69	260	
17:39	65	275	
18:41	62	290	
19:40	59	305	
20:36	56	320	
21:30	54	335	
22:21	51	350	
23:10	49	365	
23:57	47	380	
24:43	46	395	
25:27	44	410	
26:09	42	425	
26:50	41	440	
27:30	40	455	
28:08	38	470	
28:45	37	485	
29:21	36	500	
29:56	35	515	
30:30	34	530	
31:03	32	560	

Conconi's test is an excellent and simple way to test athletes. In practice, the execution of the test and the interpretation of the data are sometimes problematic, and there is considerable comment on this test in international literature.

First, in the curves of some athletes the HRdefl is not noticeable or hardly noticeable. I estimate that this occurs with 25% of tested athletes, even when the test is carried out correctly. But even when the Dp—the bend in the HR curve—cannot be determined, the test (if carried out correctly) provides ample information. Second, execution of the test takes some experience, and accuracy is vital. Such accuracy is sometimes absent in everyday practice.

I have worked with this test for some years now to my full satisfaction. Sometimes I combine the test with other methods, just to be sure of the correct HRdefl.

Finding the Deflection Point

There are many ways to find the HRdefl. The resting HR (HRrest) and HRmax methods are very easy. The flat maximum endurance effort of 30 to 60 minutes and the IAT method are suitable. Also the actual time and pace on 5 and 10 kilometers are starting points. It is not difficult or complicated for an athlete to find out his or her HRdefl or IAT. However, one laboratory test can end all doubts. It takes a well-experienced sports medicine institution to find the HRdefl or IAT by means of Conconi's test or a lactate test.

Determining the HRdefl Without Measuring Lactate

The athlete can determine his or her own HRdefl without the help of laboratories and elaborate tests. Cyclists can do this with a bicycle ergometer.

This is a simple test that provides a lot of information. The HRdefl can be estimated and will easily indicate an improvement or deterioration of condition. There is no need for a laboratory. But the test requires accuracy, so it should always be conducted under equal circumstances. This test can only be conducted when the athlete already has a fairly accurate idea of where the HRdefl is. The test is then done to verify this information.

Determining the HRdefl on a bicycle ergometer

Requirements

Ergometer that can be tuned exactly for power output

HR monitor to register the HR curve

Execution of the test

Warm up for 5 to 10 minutes.

Choose a workload that can be repeated 10 to 15 times, for example, 15 × 3 minutes at 325 watts, with always the same pedaling frequency, for example, 100 RPM.

Recovery periods are exactly 1 minute.

Keep the same pedaling frequency during the recovery periods, for example, frequency 60 RPM at 100 watts.

Keep an eye on the clock. For every next step, try to catch the rhythm of 100 RPM as fast as possible.

When the curve is plotted (see graph 64), it will be clear that HR no longer increases from a certain point; this is the HRdefl.

Determining the HRdefl on the Bike

The athlete should make a maximum effort for 30 to 60 minutes. This effort should be flat, so that the pace does not decrease by the end of the test. The HR during this effort corresponds well with the HRdefl.

Graph 65 records a maximum, flat effort during 60 minutes. This represents a cycling workout on the road with a constant high speed and average HR of 160. The HRdefl expected in this athlete is 160. In a laboratory test, the HRdefl was also 160. The test on the road shows the same HRdefl as the lactate test on an ergometer.

It is fairly simple to estimate the HRdefl with the help of an HR monitor. After a 10-minute warm-up, a constant pace is run or cycled during 10 minutes, with the HR kept constant at 140. After 10 minutes the athlete accelerates to HR 150, then 10 minutes at HR 160, and then 10 minutes at HR 170. The HR at which the 10 minutes cannot be done orcan be done only at great cost is about five beats above the HRdefl, so the HR of the last step minus five is the HRdefl. Cyclists can also perform this test on an ergometer. Graph 66 illustrates this means of determining HRdefl.

The HRdefl also can be determined by accelerating cycling speed per 10 kilometers. On a certain fixed workout route, the athlete completes four laps of 10 kilometers each. The first lap is performed at HR 145, the second at HR 155, the third at HR 165, and the last lap at HRdefl. The speed and heart rate are plotted in a curve. This curve is an excellent standard for the condition of that moment and is a practical way of estimating HRdefl. The athlete should repeat this test after a few weeks to monitor for improvement. This test is shown in graph 67.

The HRdefl and climbing capacity of a cyclist can be established very simply. The difference in altitude bridged by the rider in a certain period of time is extrapolated to an altitude difference per hour. This test supplies

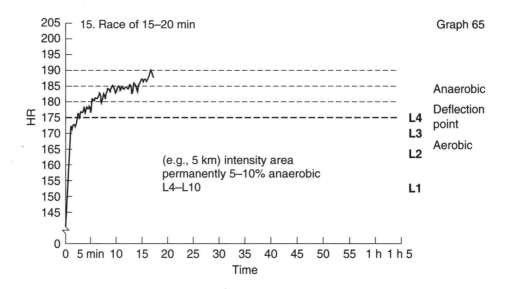

information about climbing capacity, condition, and HRdefl of the rider. When test rides are conducted regularly under nearly the same circumstances, improvement in climbing capacity and condition can be established. In addition, changes in the Dp are easily noticed. Another advantage is that the climbing capacity of riders can be compared with others. An amateur who has ambitions to become a pro may determine if he or she has a chance in that discipline among the professional riders. Graph 68 shows a plot of a climbing time trial.

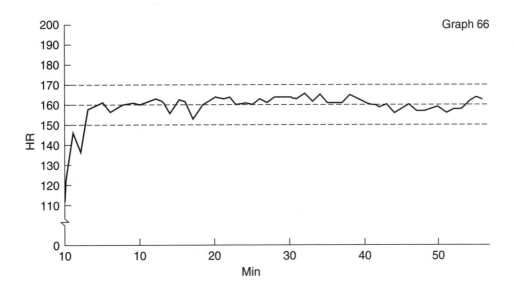

Graph 66

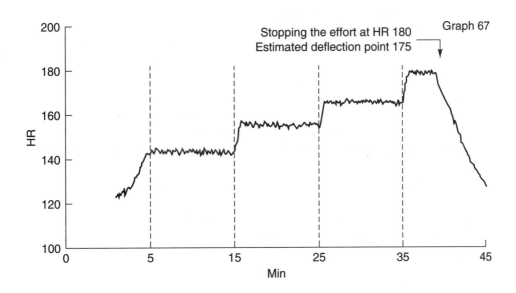

Graph 67

Stopping the effort at HR 180
Estimated deflection point 175

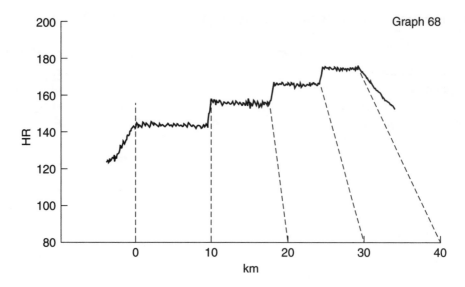

Lance Armstrong in *Sport International* stated, "In the forecast of the Tour de France of 1999 the media doubted my climbing capacities. I did not share these doubts. As a training workout we have climbed a slope in the neighborhood of Nice, on which Tony Rominger always tested himself, a couple of times. We did that with all the riders who lived in the vicinity like Axel Merckx, Bobby Julich and Kevin Livingstone. We knew what was fast. Before the Tour I did a very good test there; I was the fastest of them all. From that moment onwards I felt confident about my climbing capacities."

To execute the climbing test, the cyclist should choose an even, regular slope that requires about 30 to 45 minutes and then should ride uphill as fast as possible. Tony Rominger rode his test in Switzerland—the Col de Madone with a difference in altitude of 903 meters—in 31 minutes. With this speed he could have done 1,748 meters in 1 hour. This difference of 1,748 meters is the standard for the climbing capacity of Tony Rominger.

The best climbing capacity is that of Marco Pantani, who made 1,850 meters difference in altitude per hour on the Alpe d'Huez. The climb to the Alpe d'Huez starts at 600 meters above sea level and ends at 1,850 meters, so the difference in altitude that has to be overcome is 1,250 meters. Gert-Jan Theunisse rode the climb to the Alpe d'Huez many times. His fastest time, during the Tour de France 1988, was 00:42:50. He was second then behind Steven Rooks. The fastest time in a training workout was 00:42:03. In the race, Theunisse used the following gears: 42 × 18, 42 × 17, 42 × 16. The climbing capacity of the fastest workout was 1,783 meters.

If the athlete is unable to plot a lactate curve, the HRmax might give sufficient information. Starting from the HRmax, the various training intensities can be set accurately. The information supplied in table 3.5 only applies to well-trained cyclists. In addition, the HRmax can only be established when the rider has rested well enough.

The determination is done as follows: A 10-minute warm-up is followed by a maximum time trial effort of 3 to 4 minutes. The last 20 to 30 seconds are sprinted. The HRmax now can be read on the HR monitor. Do not use a single determination for the HRmax. More attempts, preferable also under racing conditions, are needed to accurately determine HRmax (see table 3.5).

Table 3.5		Lactate Values Deduced From HRmax for Cyclists								
HRmax	L4	L3	L2.5	L2		HRmax	L4	L3	L2.5	L2
150	137	133	129	124		180	165	159	155	149
151	138	133	130	125		181	166	160	155	150
152	139	134	131	126		182	167	161	156	150
153	140	135	131	127		183	168	162	157	151
154	141	135	132	127		184	168	163	158	152
155	142	137	133	128		185	169	163	159	153
153	143	138	134	129		186	170	164	160	154
157	144	139	135	130		187	171	165	161	155
158	145	140	136	131		188	172	166	161	155
159	146	140	137	131		189	173	167	162	156
160	147	141	137	132		190	174	168	163	157
161	147	142	138	133		191	175	169	164	158
162	148	143	139	134		192	176	170	165	159
163	149	144	140	135		193	177	171	166	160
164	150	145	141	136		194	178	171	167	160
165	151	146	142	136		195	179	172	167	161
166	152	147	143	137		196	179	173	168	162
167	153	148	143	138		197	180	174	169	163
168	154	148	144	139		198	181	175	170	164
169	155	149	145	140		199	182	176	171	165
170	156	150	146	141		200	183	177	172	165
171	157	151	147	141		201	184	178	173	166
172	158	152	148	142		202	185	178	173	167
173	158	153	149	143		203	186	179	174	168
174	159	154	149	144		204	187	180	175	169
175	160	155	150	145		205	188	181	176	170
176	161	156	151	146		206	189	182	177	170
177	162	156	152	146		207	190	183	178	181
178	163	157	153	147		208	190	184	179	172
179	164	158	154	148		209	191	185	179	173

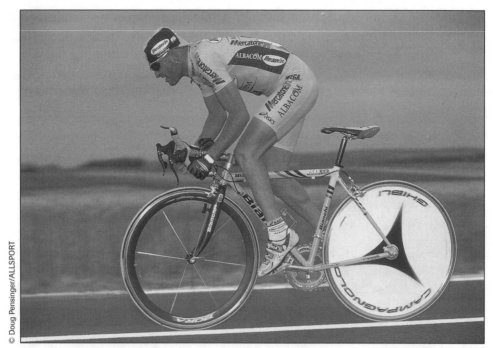

"Strong–climber" Marco Pantani, winner of the 1998 Tour de France, overcomes 1,250 meters on the Alpe d' Huez.

Individual Anaerobic Threshold Test

The IAT running test consists of five to six consecutive runs. Depending on the athlete's level of conditioning, the distances are 800, 1,000, or 1,200 meters. With an expected threshold pace between 13 and 15 kilometers per hour, the test runs are 800 meters long; at 15 to 17 kilometers per hour, the test runs are 1,000 meters long; and at 17 to 20 kilometers per hour, they are 1,200 meters long.

The test can best be done on an athletics track or a fixed route with marks at every 200 meters, because each run should be done 2 seconds faster per 200 meters than the previous one. Between every run there is a recovery pause of 50 seconds of walking. The V4 pace is reached in the fourth or fifth run. The HR corresponding to that pace is the HRdefl. Running intensities in distances from 100 meters to the marathon are related to the V4 pace.

Graph 69 shows the relationship between running intensity and distance. The V4 pace is 100%. The 5,000-meter race is run at an intensity of 109.3% and the marathon at an intensity of 94.3%. Once the V4 pace of an athlete is known, the optimal time of these distances can be calculated by using these percentages (see table 3.6).

Here are two calculation examples. First, an athlete with a known V4 pace of 16 kilometers per hour runs 1 kilometer in 00:03:45. The athlete may run an optimal marathon at 94% of V4, that is, 15 kilometers per hour, which

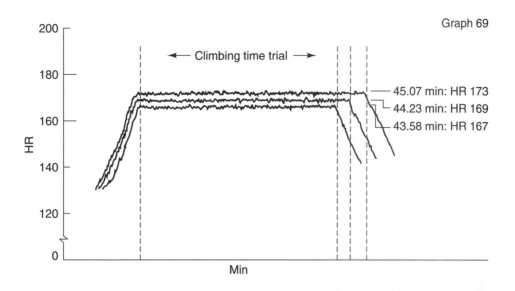

Graph 69

← Climbing time trial →

45.07 min: HR 173
44.23 min: HR 169
43.58 min: HR 167

HR

Min

Table 3.6	The V4 Pace (min:sec) Deduced From the 5K and 10K Times (min:sec)		
5K times	**V4 pace**	**10K times**	**V4 pace time/km**
22:45	5:00 (= 12 km/h)		
22:34	4:54	33:30	3:32 (= 17km/h)
22:22	4:48	32:45	3:26
21:41	4:42	32:00	3:20 (= 18 km/h)
21:00	4:37 (= 13 km/h)	31:15	3:15
21:10	4:37 (= 13 km/h)	30:30	3:10
20:52	4:33	29:45	3:05
20:34	4:29	29:00	3:00 (= 20 km/h)
20:16	4:25		
19:58	4:21		
19:40	4:17 (= 14 km/h)		
19:25	4:14		
19:10	4:10		
18:55	4:07		
18:40	4:03		
18:25	4:00 (= 15 km/h)		

(continued)

Table 3.6 *(continued)*

5K times	V4 pace	10K times	V4 pace time/km
18:16	3:57		
18:02	3:54		
17:48	3:51		
17:34	3:48		
17:20	3:45 (= 16 km/h)		
17:07	3:42		
16:54	3:40		
16:41	3:37		
16:28	3:34		
16:15	3:32 (= 17 km/h)		

Table 3.7 Intensity Table Related to the IAT

Intensity (%)		Type of workout
120	Anaerobic 1 (An1)	Short intervals
110		Intermediate intervals
103	Endurance 2 (E2)	Long intervals
100		Threshold workouts
97	Endurance 1 (E1)	High-speed endurance
95		Normal endurance
91	Aerobic 2 (A2)	Endurance at intermediate pace
85		
80	Aerobic 1 (A1)	Endurance at slow pace
75	Recovery	Recovery runs

means 1 kilometer in 00:04:00, so the athlete's marathon time will be 02:48:00. The athlete's half marathon at 98.4% of V4, that is, 15.7 kilometers per hour, is 01:20:00. On the basis of the personal best times on the 5- or 10-kilometer run, the V4 pace may be calculated. The HR corresponding to this threshold pace is the HRdefl. The V4 pace is set at 100%. Second, a runner with a time of 00:18:30 on the 5,000-meter run has a calculated V4 pace or an IAT of 4 minutes per kilometer, or 15 kilometers per hour. This athlete runs 5,000 meters at an intensity of about 109% and 10,000 meters at 104%. Tables 3.7 and 3.8 show the relationship between intensity and IAT.

An athlete who runs 5,000 meters in 00:18:30 performs six test runs of 800 or 1,000 meters. The athlete's V4 pace is 15 kilometers per hour or 4 minutes per kilometer, and the calculated IAT time per 200 meters is 48 seconds. This pace of 48 seconds per 200 meters should be reached in Run 5. Every run before that will be 2 seconds slower per 200 meters. Run 5 is 48 seconds, Run 4 is 50 seconds, Run 3 is 52 seconds, Run 2 is 54 seconds, and Run 1 is 56 seconds.

For good results, more tests should be performed under equal circumstances. It will take some time to be able to execute the test well, but the test will only be valuable when executed accurately. The athlete should start with a warm-up, immediately followed by the first run. After every run the athlete walks for 50 seconds. These recovery pauses are of major importance because the HR at the end of this pause provides the most important information of this test. Every test run should be done at the correct pace. A helper could possibly check the 200-meter times, or the athlete could use the system used for Conconi's test, where a sound signal on tape indicates the correct pace. See table 3.9.

Drawing a line through the downward tips of the recovery curve in graph 70 indicates that recovery is decreased after Run 5. The IAT of this example is between Runs 4 and 5. The estimated threshold pace at the IAT lies between 00:03:08 and 00:02:59, about 00:03:05 per 800 meters, which is 00:03:51 per 1,000 meters or 15.6 kilometers per hour. The estimated HRdefl lies between HR 165 and 173, thus HR 170. See table 3.10.

Table 3.8   Intensity

Recovery		= 70-80%	= duration 30-45 min
A1	= aerobic1	= 80-90%	= duration 50-90 min
A2	= aerobic 2	= 90-95%	= duration 30-50 min
E1	= endurance 1	= 95-100%	= duration 20-30 min
	Anaerobic threshold = 100% = deflection point = V4 pace		
E2	= endurance 2	= 100-110%	= intervals
An1	= anaerobic 1	= 110-120%	= intervals

Table 3.9   Protocol for IAT Test for Runners

Test runs: 800-1,000-1,200 m	Time sec/200 m at various threshold paces						
Threshold pace km/h	**13.0**	**14.0**	**15.0**	**16.0**	**17.0**	**18.0**	**19.0**	**20.0**
Run 1	63.5	59.5	56	53	50	48	46	44
Run 2	61.5	57.5	54	51	48	46	44	42
Run 3	59.5	55.5	52	49	46	44	42	40
Run 4	57.5	53.5	50	47	44	42	40	38
Run 5 (IAT)	55.5	51.5	48	45	42	40	38	36
Run 6	53.5	49.5	46	43	40	38	36	34

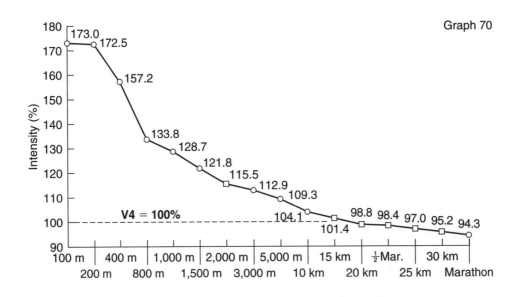

Graph 70

Table 3.10 Test Run Times and HRs

Run	Time (min:sec)	HR after recovery	HR after 50 sec
Run 1	5:19	148	122
Run 2	3:25	153	120
Run 3	3:17	160	130
Run 4	3:08	165	136
Run 5	2:59	173	146
Run 6	2:54	177	150
Run 7	1:23	170	147

Note: Data IAT test; Run 1 = 1,200 m; Runs 2-6 = 800 m; Run 7 = 400 m

Determining the HRdefl for Runners, Derived From a 1–Hour Run

Athletes who do not possess an HR monitor may use table 3.11 to find the most effective training intensity. They will need to know their V4 pace. Beside the lactate test or Conconi's test, the pace in an even 1-hour run is a reliable indication of conditioning status. See graph 71 (running intensity dependent on distance).

The formula for calculating the V4 pace is as follows:

Distance covered in meters ÷ time in seconds

For example, the distance covered in an even 1-hour run is 16,200 meters.

The V4 pace is 16,200 ÷ 3,600 = 4.50 meters per second. This corresponds with 16,200 kilometers per hour. So V4 pace is 4.50 meters per second or 16,220 kilometers per hour. This pace is the basis for determining the other training intensities. Once the HRdefl is known, the other intensities may simply be read in table 3.12.

It is well known that the marathon can be run at an intensity of about 95% of the V4 pace. In this example, the predicted marathon time would be 02:46:00. Because the values of table 3.11 depend greatly on circumstances that may change daily, they are only rough approaches. The runner of the preceding example may use 16,200 ± 400 meters. The athlete should regularly record his or her time per 200 meters during workouts. In the preceding example (15,800 to 16,600 kilometers per hour), the A1 pace in table 3.12 is between 3.51 and 3.69 meters per second.

Calculated per 200 meters:

$$200 \div 3.51 = 56.9 \text{ seconds}$$

$$200 \div 3.69 = 54.2 \text{ seconds}$$

The A1 pace is between these values, and the same formula may be used for the other intensity levels. Table 3.13 shows the internationally recognized intensity levels.

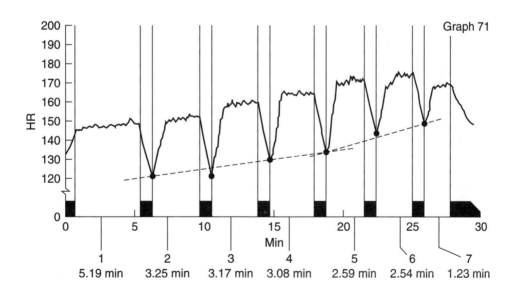

Table 3.11   For Runners (m/sec)

Anaerobic area					Deflection (km/h)		Aerobic area E1		A2	Recovery A1	RC	Marathon time (min)
125%	120%	115%	110%	103%	100%	100%	97%	95%	91%	80%	75%	
3.82	3.67	3.51	3.36	3.15	11.000	3.06	2.96	2.90	2.78	2.44	2.29	244
3.89	3.73	3.58	3.42	3.20	11.200	3.11	3.02	2.96	2.83	2.49	2.33	240
3.96	3.80	3.64	3.48	3.26	11.400	3.17	3.07	3.01	2.88	2.53	2.38	236
4.03	3.87	3.71	3.54	3.32	11.600	3.22	3.13	3.06	2.93	2.58	2.42	231
4.10	3.93	3.77	3.61	3.38	11.800	3.28	3.18	3.11	2.98	2.62	2.46	288
4.17	4.00	3.83	3.67	3.43	12.000	3.33	3.23	3.17	3.03	2.67	2.50	224
4.24	4.07	3.90	3.73	3.49	12.200	3.39	3.29	3.22	3.08	2.71	2.54	220
4.31	4.13	3.96	3.79	3.55	12.400	3.44	3.34	3.27	3.13	2.76	2.58	217
4.38	4.20	4.03	3.85	3.61	12.600	3.50	3.40	3.33	3.19	2.80	2.63	213
4.44	4.27	4.09	3.91	3.66	12.800	3.56	3.45	3.38	3.24	2.84	2.67	210
4.51	4.33	4.15	3.97	3.72	13.000	3.61	3.50	3.43	3.29	2.89	2.71	207
4.58	4.40	4.22	4.03	3.78	13.200	3.67	3.56	3.48	3.34	2.93	2.75	203
4.65	4.47	4.28	4.09	3.83	13.400	3.72	3.61	3.54	3.39	2.98	3.79	200
4.72	4.53	4.34	4.16	3.89	13.600	3.78	3.66	3.59	3.44	3.02	2.83	197
4.79	4.60	4.41	4.22	3.95	13.800	3.83	3.72	3.64	3.49	3.07	2.88	195
4.86	4.67	4.47	4.28	4.01	14.000	3.89	3.77	3.69	3.54	3.11	2.92	192
4.93	4.73	4.54	4.34	4.06	14.200	3.94	3.83	3.75	3.59	3.16	2.96	189
5.00	4.80	4.60	4.40	4.12	14.400	4.00	3.88	3.80	3.64	3.20	3.00	186
5.07	4.87	4.66	4.46	4.18	14.600	4.06	3.93	3.85	3.69	3.24	3.04	184
5.14	4.93	4.73	4.52	4.23	14.800	4.11	3.99	3.91	3.74	3.29	3.08	181
5.21	5.00	4.79	4.58	4.29	15.000	4.17	4.04	3.96	3.79	3.33	3.13	179
5.28	5.07	4.86	4.64	4.35	15.200	4.22	4.10	4.01	3.84	3.38	3.17	177
5.35	5.13	4.92	4.71	4.41	15.400	4.28	4.15	4.06	3.89	3.42	3.21	174
5.42	5.20	4.98	4.77	4.46	15.600	4.33	4.20	4.12	3.94	3.47	3.25	172
5.49	5.27	5.05	4.83	4.52	15.800	4.39	4.26	4.17	3.99	3.51	3.29	170
5.56	5.33	5.11	4.89	4.58	16.000	4.44	4.31	4.22	4.04	3.56	3.33	168
5.63	5.40	5.18	4.95	4.64	16.200	4.50	4.36	4.28	4.10	3.60	3.38	166
5.69	5.47	5.24	5.01	4.69	16.400	4.56	4.42	4.33	4.15	3.64	3.42	164
5.76	5.53	5.30	5.07	4.75	16.600	4.61	4.47	4.38	4.20	3.69	3.46	162
5.83	5.60	5.37	5.13	4.81	16800	4.67	4.53	4.43	4.25	3.73	3.50	160
5.90	5.67	5.43	5.19	4.86	17.000	4.72	4.58	4.49	4.30	3.78	3.54	158
5.97	5.73	5.49	5.26	4.92	17.200	4.78	4.63	4.54	4.35	3.82	3.58	156
6.04	5.80	5.56	5.32	4.98	17.400	4.83	4.69	4.59	4.40	3.87	3.63	154
6.11	5.87	5.62	5.38	5.04	17.600	4.89	4.74	4.64	4.45	3.91	3.67	153

Anaerobic area					Deflection (km/h)		Aerobic area E1		A2	Recovery A1	RC	Marathon time (min)
125%	120%	115%	110%	103%	100%	100%	97%	95%	91%	80%	75%	
6.18	5.93	5.69	5.44	5.09	17.800	4.94	4.80	4.70	4.50	3.96	3.71	151
6.25	6.00	5.75	5.50	5.15	18.000	5.00	4.85	4.75	4.55	4.00	3.75	149
6.32	6.07	5.81	5.56	5.21	18.200	5.06	4.90	4.80	4.60	4.04	3.79	148
6.39	6.13	5.88	5.62	5.26	18.400	5.11	4.96	4.86	4.65	4.09	3.83	146
6.46	6.20	5.94	5.68	5.32	18.600	5.17	5.01	4.91	4.70	4.13	3.88	144
6.53	6.27	6.01	5.74	5.38	18.800	5.22	5.07	4.96	4.75	4.18	3.93	143
6.60	6.33	6.07	5.81	5.44	19.000	5.28	5.12	5.01	4.80	4.22	3.96	141
6.67	6.40	6.13	5.87	5.49	19.200	5.33	5.17	5.07	4.85	4.27	4.00	140
6.74	6.47	6.20	5.93	5.55	19.400	5.39	5.23	5.12	4.90	4.31	4.04	138
6.81	6.53	6.26	5.99	5.61	19.600	5.44	5.28	5.17	4.95	4.36	4.08	137
6.88	6.60	6.33	6.05	4.67	19.800	5.50	5.34	5.23	5.01	4.40	4.13	136
6.94	6.67	6.39	6.11	5.72	20.000	5.56	5.39	5.28	5.06	4.44	4.17	134
7.01	6.73	6.45	6.17	5.78	20.200	5.61	5.44	5.33	5.11	4.49	4.21	133
7.08	6.80	6.52	6.23	5.84	20.400	5.67	5.50	5.38	5.16	4.53	4.25	132
7.15	6.87	6.58	6.29	5.89	20.600	5.72	5.55	5.44	5.21	4.58	4.29	130
7.22	6.93	6.64	6.36	5.95	20.800	5.78	5.60	5.49	5.26	4.62	4.33	129
7.29	7.00	6.71	6.42	6.01	21.000	5.83	5.66	5.54	5.31	4.67	4.38	128

Table 3.12 Intensity Table for Runners Calculated in Meters per Second

Anaerobic area					Deflection V4		Anaerobic area E1		A2	Recovery A1	RC	Marathon time (min)
125%	120%	115%	110%	103%	100%	100%	97%	95%	91%	80%	75%	
4.22	4.33	4.45	4.58	5.18	11.000	5.27	5.37	5.44	6.00	6.59	7.16	244
4.17	4.28	4.40	4.52	5.12	11.200	5.21	5.31	5.38	5.53	6.42	7.09	240
4.13	4.23	4.35	4.47	5.07	11.400	5.16	5.26	5.32	5.47	6.35	7.01	236
4.08	4.19	4.30	4.42	5.01	11.600	5.10	5.20	5.27	5.41	6.28	6.54	231
4.04	4.14	4.25	4.37	4.56	11.800	5.05	5.15	5.21	5.35	6.21	6.47	288
4.00	4.10	4.21	4.33	4.51	12.000	5.00	5.09	5.16	5.30	6.15	6.40	224
3.56	4.06	4.17	4.28	4.46	12.200	4.55	5.04	5.11	5.24	6.09	6.33	220
3.52	4.02	4.12	4.24	4.42	12.400	4.50	4.59	5.06	5.19	6.03	6.27	217
3.49	3.58	4.08	4.20	4.37	12.600	4.46	4.55	5.01	5.14	5.57	6.21	213
3.45	3.54	4.05	4.16	4.33	12.800	4.41	4.50	4.56	5.09	5.52	6.15	210
3.42	3.51	4.01	4.12	4.29	13.000	4.37	4.45	4.51	5.04	5.46	6.09	207

(continued)

Table 3.12 *(continued)*

Anaerobic area					Deflection V4		Anaerobic area E1		A2	Recovery A1	RC	Marathon time (min)
125%	120%	115%	110%	103%	100%	100%	97%	95%	91%	80%	75%	
3.38	3.47	3.57	4.08	4.25	13.200	4.33	4.41	4.47	5.00	5.41	6.04	203
3.35	3.44	3.54	4.04	4.21	13.400	4.29	4.37	4.43	4.55	5.36	5.58	200
3.32	3.41	3.50	4.01	4.17	13.600	4.25	4.33	4.39	4.51	5.31	5.53	197
3.29	3.37	3.47	3.57	4.13	13.800	4.21	4.29	4.35	4.47	5.26	5.48	195
3.26	3.34	3.44	3.54	4.10	14.000	4.17	4.25	4.31	4.43	5.21	5.43	192
3.23	3.31	3.40	3.50	4.06	14.200	4.14	4.21	4.27	4.39	5.17	5.38	189
3.20	3.28	3.37	3.47	4.03	14.000	4.10	4.18	4.23	4.35	5.13	5.33	186
3.17	3.25	3.34	3.44	3.59	14.600	4.07	4.14	4.20	4.31	5.08	5.29	184
3.15	3.23	3.32	3.41	3.56	14.800	4.03	4.11	4.16	4.27	5.04	5.24	181
3.12	3.20	3.29	3.38	3.53	15.000	4.00	4.07	4.13	4.24	5.00	5.20	179
3.09	3.17	3.26	3.35	3.50	15.200	3.57	4.04	4.09	4.20	4.56	5.16	177
3.07	3.15	3.23	3.33	3.47	15.400	3.54	4.01	4.06	4.17	4.52	5.12	174
3.05	3.12	3.21	3.30	3.44	15.600	3.51	3.58	4.03	4.14	4.48	5.08	172
3.02	3.10	3.18	3.27	3.41	15.800	3.48	3.55	4.00	4.10	4.45	5.04	170
3.00	3.08	3.16	3.25	3.38	16.000	3.45	3.52	3.57	4.07	4.41	5.00	168
2.58	3.05	3.13	3.22	3.36	16.200	3.42	3.49	3.54	4.04	4.38	4.56	166
2.56	3.03	3.11	3.20	3.33	16.400	3.40	3.46	3.51	4.01	4.34	4.53	164
2.53	3.01	3.09	3.17	3.31	16.600	3.37	3.44	3.48	3.58	4.31	4.49	162
3.51	2.59	3.06	3.15	3.28	16.800	3.34	3.41	3.46	3.55	3.28	4.46	160
2.49	2.56	3.04	3.13	3.26	17.000	3.32	3.38	3.43	3.53	4.25	4.42	158
2.47	2.54	3.02	3.10	3.23	17.200	3.29	3.36	3.40	3.50	4.22	4.39	156
2.46	2.52	3.00	3.08	3.21	17.400	3.27	3.33	3.38	3.47	4.19	4.36	154
2.44	2.50	2.58	3.06	3.19	17.600	3.25	3.31	3.35	3.45	4.16	4.33	153
2.42	2.49	2.56	3.04	3.16	17.800	3.22	3.29	3.33	3.42	4.13	4.30	151
2.40	2.47	2.54	3.02	3.14	18.000	3.20	3.26	3.31	3.40	4.10	4.27	149
2.38	2.45	2.52	3.00	3.12	18.200	3.18	3.24	3.28	3.37	4.07	4.24	148
2.37	2.43	2.50	2.58	3.10	18.400	3.16	3.22	3.26	3.35	4.05	4.21	146
2.35	2.41	2.48	2.56	3.08	18.600	3.14	3.20	3.24	3.33	4.02	4.18	144
2.33	2.40	2.47	2.54	3.06	18.800	3.11	3.17	3.22	3.30	3.59	4.15	143
2.32	2.38	2.45	2.52	3.04	19.000	3.09	3.15	3.19	3.28	3.57	4.13	141

Anaerobic area					Deflection V4		Anaerobic area E1		A2	Recovery A1	RC	Marathon time (min)
125%	120%	115%	110%	103%	100%	100%	97%	95%	91%	80%	75%	
2.30	2.36	2.43	2.50	3.02	19.200	3.08	3.13	3.17	3.26	3.54	4.10	140
2.28	2.35	2.41	2.49	3.00	19.400	3.06	3.11	3.15	3.24	3.52	4.07	138
2.27	2.33	2.40	2.47	2.58	19.600	3.04	3.09	3.13	3.22	3.50	4.05	137
2.25	2.32	2.38	2.45	2.57	19.800	3.02	3.07	3.11	3.20	3.47	4.02	136
2.24	2.30	2.37	2.44	2.55	20.000	3.00	3.06	3.09	3.18	3.45	4.00	134
2.23	2.29	2.35	2.42	2.53	20.200	2.58	3.04	3.08	3.16	3.43	3.58	133
2.21	2.27	2.33	2.40	2.51	20.400	2.56	3.02	3.06	3.14	3.41	3.55	132
2.20	2.26	2.32	2.39	2.50	20.600	2.55	3.00	3.04	3.12	3.38	3.53	130
2.18	2.24	2.31	2.37	2.48	20.800	2.53	2.58	3.02	3.10	3.36	3.51	129
2.17	2.23	2.29	2.36	2.46	21.000	2.51	2.57	3.00	3.08	3.34	3.49	128

Table 3.13 Intensity Table for Runners, Derived From Personal Best Time on 10km V4

Best time 10K (min:sec)	Pace 10K (km/h)	Threshold pace (km/h)	Threshold pace (min:sec)	Marathon pace (km/h)	Marathon pace (h:min)
29:00	20.7	19.9	3:01	18.7	2:15
29:30	20.3	19.6	3:04	18.4	2:18
30:00	20.0	19.2	3:07	18.0	2:20
30:30	19.7	18.9	3:10	17.8	2:23
31:00	19.4	18.6	3:13	17.5	2:25
31:30	19.0	18.3	3:17	17.2	2:27
32:00	18.7	18.0	3:20	16.9	2:30
33:00	18.2	17.5	3:26	16.4	2:36
34:00	17.6	16.9	3:32	15.9	2:39
35:00	17.1	16.5	3:38	15.5	2:43
36:00	16.6	16.0	3:45	15.1	2:48
37:00	16.2	15.6	3:51	14.7	2:53
38:00	15.8	15.2	3:57	14.3	2:58
39:00	15.4	14.8	4:03	13.9	3:02
40:00	15.0	14.4	4:10	13.6	3:07

Determining HRdefl for Runners, Deduced From the Best Time on 10 Kilometers

As an example, an athlete's best 10-kilometer time 30 minutes. The athlete's pace is 20 kilometers per hour. The 10-kilometer race is run with an intensity of 104% of the V4 pace. The V4 pace (which is put at 100%) now can be calculated easily; it is 19.2 kilometers per hour. On the basis of this V4 pace, the other training and race intensities may be read. (See table 3.14) The personal best times on 5,000 meters, 15,000 meters, and 21,000 meters can be used as well.

There is a fixed relationship between HRdefl and the other training intensities. Once the individual HRdefl (HR at a lactate level of 4 millimoles per liter, or L4) is known, the other training intensities can be found with the help of the HR table for runners.

In the example we start from an HRdefl of 175 = L4. The other intensities can be read in table 3.14 (L3, L2.5, L2, and L1). The characteristic HR curves are shown in graphs 72 through 88B.

Table 3.14   HR/ Lactate for Runners

HR/L4	HR/L3	HR/L2.5	HR/L2	HR/L1	HR/L4	HR/L3	HR/L2.5	HR/L2	HR/L1
140	137	134	132	122	171	167	164	162	149
141	138	135	133	122	172	168	165	163	149
142	139	136	134	123	173	169	166	164	150
143	140	137	135	124	174	170	167	164	151
144	141	138	136	125	175	171	168	165	152
145	142	139	137	126	176	172	169	166	153
146	142	140	138	127	177	173	170	167	154
147	143	141	139	128	178	174	171	168	155
148	144	142	140	129	179	175	172	169	156
149	145	143	141	129	180	178	173	170	156
150	146	144	142	130	181	177	174	171	157
151	147	145	143	131	182	178	175	172	158
152	148	146	144	132	183	179	176	173	159
153	149	147	145	133	184	180	177	174	160
154	150	148	146	134	185	181	178	175	161
155	151	149	147	135	186	182	179	176	162
156	152	150	147	136	187	183	180	177	163
157	153	151	148	136	188	183	180	178	163
158	154	152	149	137	189	184	181	179	164
159	155	153	150	138	190	185	182	180	165

HR/L4	HR/L3	HR/L2.5	HR/L2	HR/L1	HR/L4	HR/L3	HR/L2.5	HR/L2	HR/L1
160	156	154	151	139	191	186	183	181	166
161	157	155	152	140	192	187	184	181	167
162	158	156	153	141	193	188	185	182	168
163	159	156	154	142	194	189	186	163	169
164	160	157	155	142	195	190	187	184	170
165	161	158	156	143	196	191	188	185	170
166	162	159	157	144	197	192	189	186	171
167	163	160	158	145	198	193	190	187	172
168	164	161	159	146	199	194	191	188	173
169	165	162	160	147	200	195	192	189	174
170	166	163	161	148					

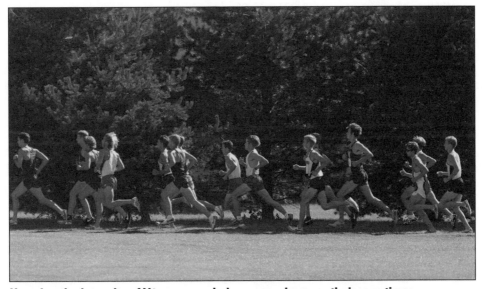

Knowing the intensity of V4 pace can help runners improve their race times.

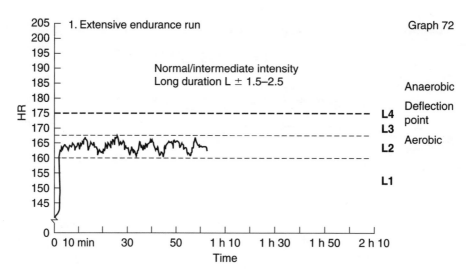

1. Extensive endurance run

Graph 72

Normal/intermediate intensity
Long duration L ± 1.5–2.5

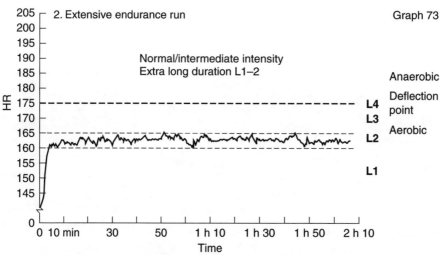

2. Extensive endurance run

Graph 73

Normal/intermediate intensity
Extra long duration L1–2

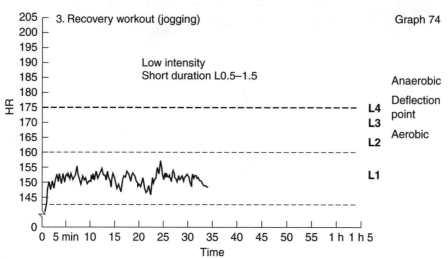

3. Recovery workout (jogging)

Graph 74

Low intensity
Short duration L0.5–1.5

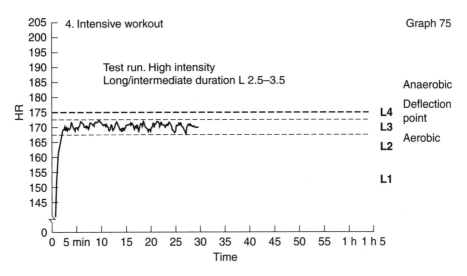

4. Intensive workout — Graph 75

Test run. High intensity
Long/intermediate duration L 2.5–3.5

Anaerobic
Deflection point
Aerobic

L4
L3
L2
L1

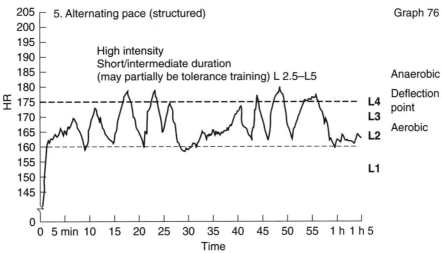

5. Alternating pace (structured) — Graph 76

High intensity
Short/intermediate duration
(may partially be tolerance training) L 2.5–L5

Anaerobic
Deflection point
Aerobic

L4
L3
L2
L1

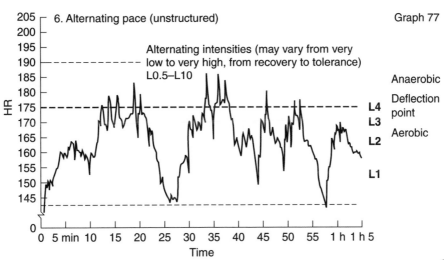

6. Alternating pace (unstructured) — Graph 77

Alternating intensities (may vary from very
low to very high, from recovery to tolerance)
L0.5–L10

Anaerobic
Deflection point
Aerobic

L4
L3
L2
L1

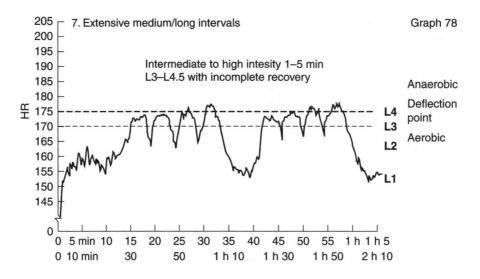

7. Extensive medium/long intervals — Graph 78

Intermediate to high intesity 1–5 min
L3–L4.5 with incomplete recovery

Anaerobic
Deflection point
Aerobic

L4
L3
L2
L1

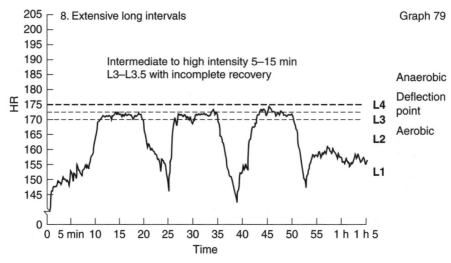

8. Extensive long intervals — Graph 79

Intermediate to high intensity 5–15 min
L3–L3.5 with incomplete recovery

Anaerobic
Deflection point
Aerobic

L4
L3
L2
L1

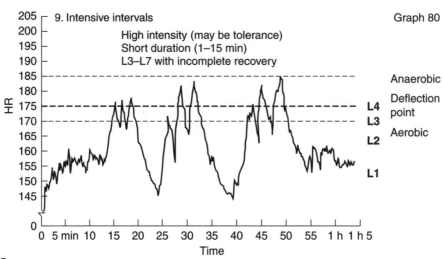

9. Intensive intervals — Graph 80

High intensity (may be tolerance)
Short duration (1–15 min)
L3–L7 with incomplete recovery

Anaerobic
Deflection point
Aerobic

L4
L3
L2
L1

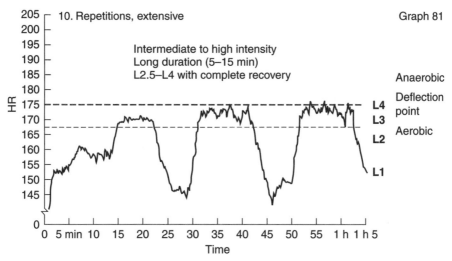

10. Repetitions, extensive — Graph 81

Intermediate to high intensity
Long duration (5–15 min)
L2.5–L4 with complete recovery

Anaerobic

Deflection point

Aerobic

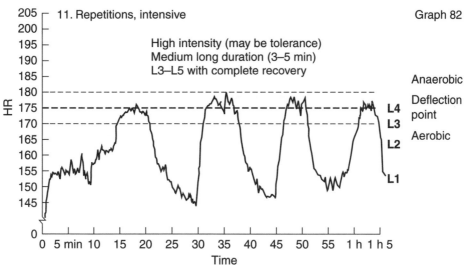

11. Repetitions, intensive — Graph 82

High intensity (may be tolerance)
Medium long duration (3–5 min)
L3–L5 with complete recovery

Anaerobic

Deflection point

Aerobic

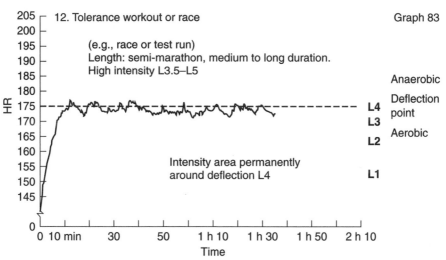

12. Tolerance workout or race — Graph 83

(e.g., race or test run)
Length: semi-marathon, medium to long duration.
High intensity L3.5–L5

Anaerobic

Deflection point

Aerobic

Intensity area permanently
around deflection L4

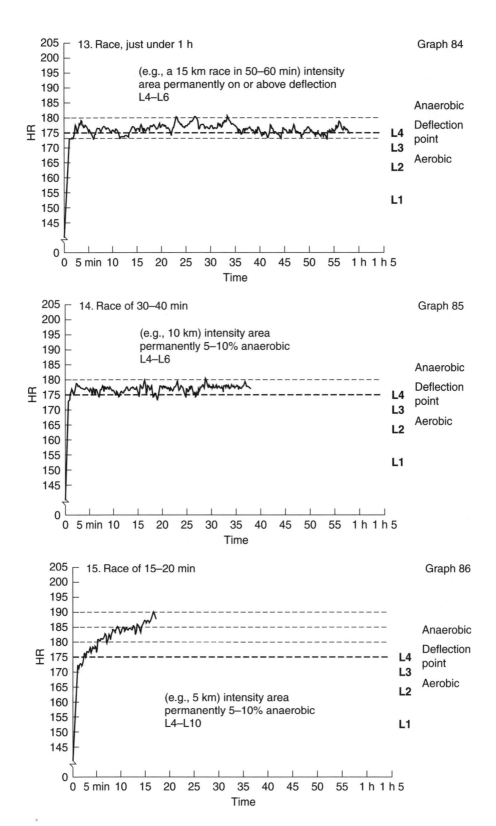

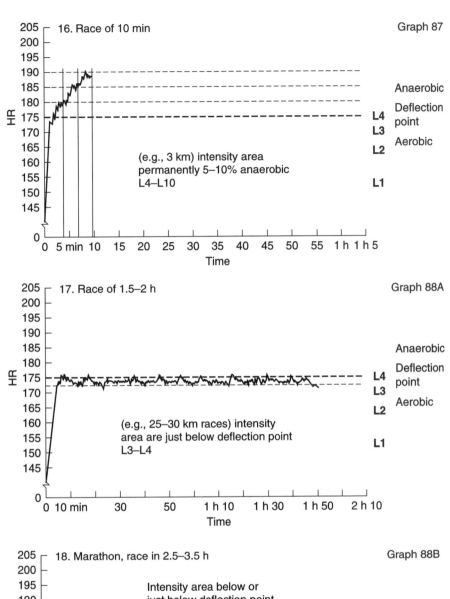

16. Race of 10 min   Graph 87

Anaerobic

Deflection point

L4
L3

Aerobic

L2

(e.g., 3 km) intensity area
permanently 5–10% anaerobic
L4–L10   L1

17. Race of 1.5–2 h   Graph 88A

Anaerobic

Deflection
point

L4
L3

Aerobic

L2

(e.g., 25–30 km races) intensity
area are just below deflection point
L3–L4   L1

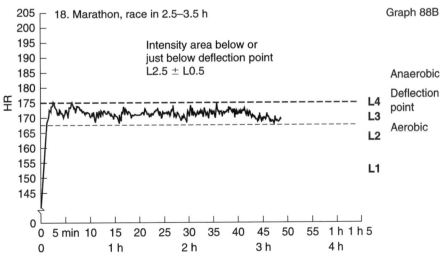

18. Marathon, race in 2.5–3.5 h   Graph 88B

Intensity area below or
just below deflection point
L2.5 ± L0.5

Anaerobic

Deflection
point

L4
L3

Aerobic

L2

L1

chapter 4

Lactate

The lactate content of the blood is a parameter of great importance. This content is measured in millimoles of lactate per liter of blood. Healthy persons at rest have values roughly between 1 and 2 millimoles per liter, and strenuous exercise increases this value. Even slight increases in lactate content (6 to 8 millimoles per liter) may impair an athlete's coordination. Regularly high lactate values impair aerobic endurance capacity.

The Lactate Curve

For this reason, athletes should be prudent with the number of intensive workloads they undergo in a certain period of time. The workload intensities needed for various workouts can be determined by means of the lactate curve. Graph 89 shows the relationship between lactate content of the blood and the intensity of exercise. Intensity is expressed as running pace in meters per second.

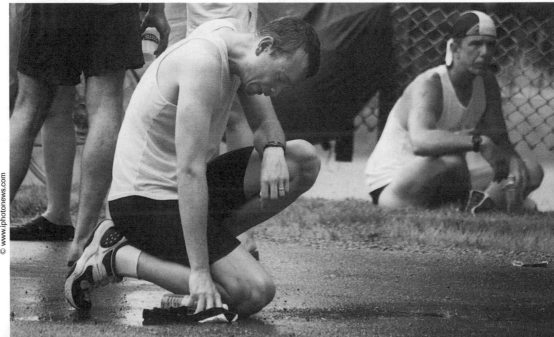

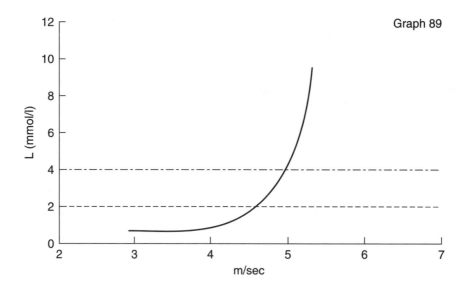

Graph 89

To obtain a lactate curve, the athlete should run the same distance a number of times, each time at a higher pace. After every run, determine the lactate concentration in the blood. Every distance should be run at an even pace, and the running pace should be increased in small steps. The length of the run should be such that the athlete needs at least 5 minutes to cover the distance. When well-trained athletes run slowly, they have low lactate values; their energy supplies are fully aerobic. When the pace is increased, the curve begins to rise; the working muscles do produce lactate, but the quantities are so small that, for the most part, they can be neutralized by the body. It is a widespread belief that this is the case between 2 and 4 millimoles per liter. Therefore, this area is called the aerobic-anaerobic transition zone.

Each athlete can maintain a certain running pace for a long period of time without lactate accumulation in the body. If the pace is increased to a certain point, ongoing acidosis will occur, depending on the degree and duration of the increase, and at a certain moment this acidosis will force the athlete to stop. The lactate content that is measured at this borderline pace is also called the anaerobic threshold. The anaerobic threshold value is around a lactate content of 4 millimoles per liter. Exercise surpassing the anaerobic threshold will inevitably increase lactate content within the body.

Thus, exercise up to this level of the aerobic threshold is fully aerobic. Lactate content at the aerobic threshold is about 2 millimoles per liter. Exercise within the aerobic-anaerobic transition zone is more intensive, and energy supply is both aerobic and anaerobic. Production and neutralization of lactate are balanced. This zone is between 2 and 4 millimoles per liter.

The anaerobic threshold occurs when exercise at a high intensity results in an accumulation of lactate in the blood. Therefore, this type of exercise can be maintained for a limited period of time. But at an intensity just below the anaerobic threshold, this lactate content can be kept at a steady-state level, and this type of exercise may be maintained for a longer period of time, about 1 to 1.5 hours.

Lactate content at the anaerobic threshold is for many athletes about 4 millimoles per liter, but there are wide individual variations among athletes. Anaerobic threshold can be as low as 2 to 3 millimoles per liter or as high as 6 to 8 millimoles per liter. By drawing a lactate curve for every athlete, the anaerobic threshold can be found and subsequently used to set training intensities. The best way to find the anaerobic threshold is to determine maximal lactate steady state (MLSS), which is discussed elsewhere in the book.

Endurance capacity can best be trained by endurance workouts around the level of the anaerobic threshold, that is, workouts with lactate values of 2 to 6 millimoles per liter. These values may be determined according to the athlete's test results. Very well-trained people mostly train their endurance capacity at somewhat lower values, between 2 and 3 millimoles per liter. Less well-trained persons often cannot help but peak to higher levels. They then surpass their anaerobic threshold and make their workouts less effective. Though they often feel satisfied with a strenuous workout, this type of workout does more damage than good.

The threshold pace is the speed that corresponds with the anaerobic threshold. Above the anaerobic threshold this speed can be maintained for a short period of time, but below the threshold it can be maintained 1 to 1.5 hours. The threshold pace, the running or cycling speed at the heart rate deflection point (HRdefl), is also called the V4 pace, as discussed in chapter 3. However, the term V4 is somewhat misleading, because many athletes have an anaerobic threshold over or under 4 millimoles per liters. For example, an athlete with an anaerobic threshold of 6 millimoles per liter could be said to have a threshold pace of V6.

Sport-specific performance capacity could be defined as the speed that is reached at a lactate content of 4 millimoles per liter, or V4. V4 is an important indicator of the athlete's capacities. Any improvement of V4 pace will also improve performance capacity. Regular V4 tests indicate the athlete's condition, so athletes can be monitored in their development and can be mutually compared. But remember that V4 is not the threshold pace for everybody, because many athletes have an anaerobic threshold under or over 4 millimoles per liter. Therefore, it might be better to test MLSS than V4.

Recovery workouts should not be intensive, and lactate content should remain less than 2 millimoles per liter. Intensive interval workouts give high lactate values, far surpassing 4 millimoles per liter. The effect of training will be that the lactate curve shifts to the right, as shown in graph 90.

Therefore, training intensities should be readjusted from time to time, and a new test procedure with blood sampling will be necessary. Not every athlete has access to blood testing, but other methods can supply the same

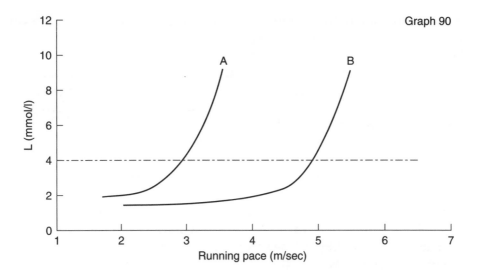

or at least the most important information. All these other methods of finding the anaerobic threshold are discussed elsewhere in this book.

Graph 91 shows lactate curves of various excellently trained athletes. Every person has a different curve, and the differences among them are often rather large. If the athlete with the curve at the extreme right trains together with the athlete whose curve is at the left and the two of them are told to perform at a heart rate (HR) of 150 beats per minute (bpm), the athlete at the left will undergo an utterly intensive workout with high lactate values, whereas the athlete at the right will hardly exert any effort. Thus, training intensities should be assessed individually. When athletes train in a group, the same workout task will be different for every athlete.

Graph 92 shows an equal effort of two athletes of the same age. The form of the two curves is almost the same, although the HR varies widely. An HR

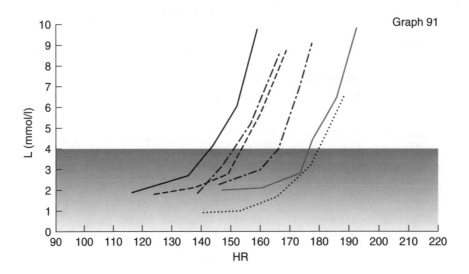

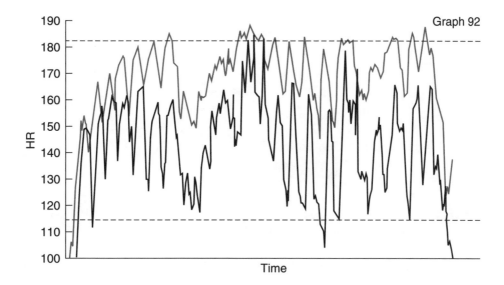

Graph 92

of 180 in the higher curve corresponds with an HR of 160 in the lower curve. Thus, these athletes are exerting an equal effort with a difference in HR of 20 bpm.

Fascinating individual differences in aerobic endurance capacity have been measured. It is clear that sprinters have lower and whole distance runners have higher aerobic capacity.

The higher the pace at a lactate content of 4 millimoles per liter, the better aerobic capacity is. Graph 93 (page 112) shows the differences in performance among a world champion pro cyclist, a world champion amateur cyclist, and a normal untrained person. The pro cyclist's maximum capacity is 430 watts, the amateur cyclist reaches 350 watts, and the untrained person reaches 190 watts. The enormous difference between the top athlete and the untrained person is accounted for by the tremendous capacity of the athlete's heart, which can circulate as much as 40 liters of blood per minute during maximum effort, whereas the untrained person's heart may reach only 20 liters per minute. Another major factor is that the top athlete's muscles can efficiently use the large amounts of oxygen delivered to them. In other words, the muscles have a large aerobic capacity.

Blood Lactate Measurement

For this method, the lactate content of the blood is measured after increasing workloads. On average, the anaerobic threshold corresponds with a blood lactate concentration of 4 millimoles per liter. But in very well-trained endurance athletes, this may be somewhat lower or in some cases higher—for example, a lactate concentration of 3 to 6 millimoles per liter. This should certainly be taken into account in planning training programs, so intensity is not too high.

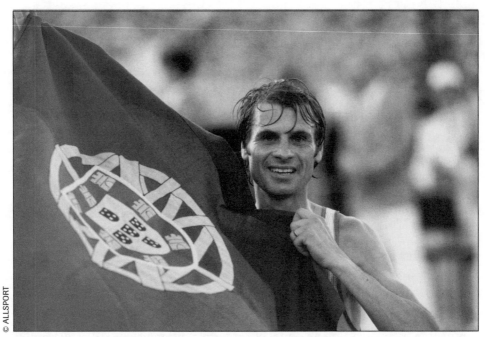

Carlos Lopes was 38 years old when he set the world record as World Cross-Country Champion and 10K Silver Olympic medalist.

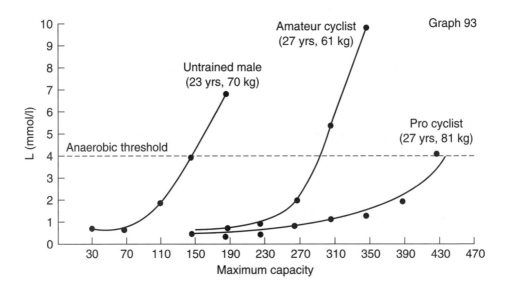

The lactate/HR curve will indicate at what HR training should be done to get an optimum effect (see graphs 94 through 96).

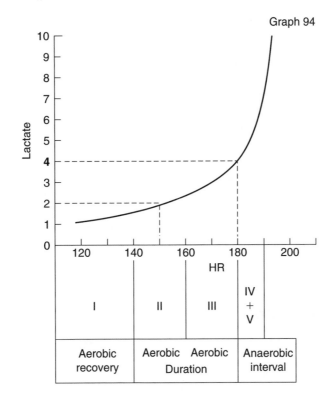

Graph 94

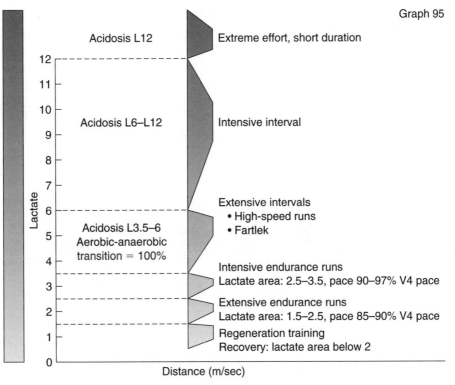

Graph 95

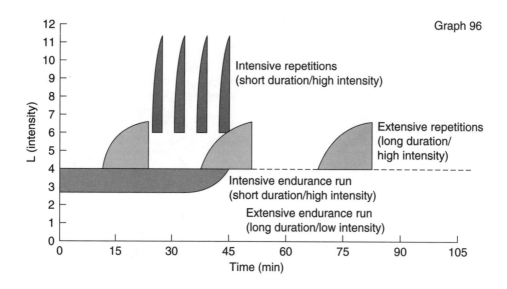

Graph 96

The Bicycle Ergometer Test

For this test the athlete starts with a 10-minute warm-up. After that, the cycling workload is increased every 5 minutes. After every 5 minutes, a 2-milliliter blood sample is taken and the HR is recorded (see table 4.1). The workload is a known factor. The test is a maximal test; the cyclist is required to exert maximal effort.

Because the cyclist rides constantly, there are no pauses for taking blood samples. Blood is drawn from a small plastic tube that is inserted in a vein in the arm before the test. During the test, blood can be taken at any moment. This blood is mixed with a test liquid in a tube, and the tubes are immediately cooled and kept on ice. The blood is centrifuged within 4 hours, separating blood cells and plasma. The plasma is placed in another tube, and this sample may be kept in a refrigerator for about 1 week. Lactate concentration of the plasma sample can now be determined by using the Boehringer method. In addition, there are now excellent portable lactate meters, with which lactate concentration can be measured immediately during the test.

Table 4.1	Determining the Anaerobic Threshold on the Bicycle Ergometer			
		HR	**W**	**L**
Warm-up	10 min	......	......	......
	15 min	......	......	......
	20 min	......	......	......

Field Test

After the athlete warms up for 10 minutes, certain distances are covered (e.g., by running, cycling, cross-country skiing, or swimming) that require a duration of 5 minutes. The athlete performs the first 5-minute segment at a low intensity. Pace is increased during the next 5-minute segment, although within each segment, the pace is kept constant and there is no final sprint. After every 5-minute period, there is a 10-minute recovery pause. The time of the last 1,000 meters in every segment and the corresponding HR are recorded, and a 2-milliliter blood sample is taken after every segment (see table 4.2). The number of meters per second can now easily be calculated.

Table 4.2 Determining the Anaerobic Threshold in a Field Test				
Warm-up (10 min)	**Time (1,000 m)**	**m/sec**	**HR**	**L**
1st 5 min				
10-min recovery				
2nd 5 min				
10-min recovery				
3rd 5 min				
10-min recovery				
4th 5 min				

Requirements for the ergometer test and the field test

- Bicycle ergometer
- HR monitor
- Materials to take blood samples
- Centrifuge
- Cooler to keep blood samples on ice
- Test protocol
- Laboratory facilities for lactate determination or portable lactate meter
- For the field test: a route

For a reliable test, the athlete should observe the following guidelines:

- Always perform the test under the same circumstances and at the same time of day.
- Do not eat a substantial meal in the 5 hours before the test.
- Abstain from alcohol for 24 hours before the test.
- Get a good night's sleep.
- Abstain from coffee, tea, or other caffeine in the last hour before the test.
- Do not train or do heavy physical work on the day of the test.
- Do not train too strenuously the day before the test.
- Always test in a constant temperature and air humidity.
- Do not perform the test when ill or feverish.
- Always warm up sufficiently before the test.

In the Laboratory

The anaerobic threshold may be determined in various ways but is generally determined in a laboratory. Some coaches believe that sport-specific testing is more accurate, and there are simple Conconi tests for the athletics track, the bicycle ergometer, or the treadmill; however, laboratory tests can be standardized better than field tests. During the test, the exercise is made more and more strenuous and a blood sample is taken at certain times for lactate determination. HR is recorded during the complete test. The curve showing the relationship between HR and lactate concentration can now easily be constructed.

Graphs 97 and 98 show the data from an exertion test with increasing workloads. Just before the workload is increased, a blood sample is taken for lactate determination. The HR is measured continually. Under the curve in graph 97 are the HR and lactate concentration that correspond with each other. The data of the curve are worked out in a lactate–HR graph (see graph 98). From this graph the HR–lactate relationship can now be read.

Graph 99 shows a different method of determining anaerobic threshold in the laboratory. This athlete's anaerobic threshold is determined by having him cycle 10 watts more every 6 minutes. Lactate is determined every third and sixth minute.

At 290 watts, lactate content does not increase, but at 300 watts, it does. So the anaerobic threshold is reached at a workload of 290 watts. The lactate or anaerobic threshold can be expressed in running pace, in cycling speed (i.e., on a sheltered track), in HR, or in watts. Once the HR of the anaerobic threshold is determined, each workout can be assessed with the help of an HR monitor.

For good endurance athletes, the anaerobic threshold is as close as possible to the maximal oxygen uptake ($\dot{V}O_2$max). Elite marathon runners can perform at 95% of their $\dot{V}O_2$max.

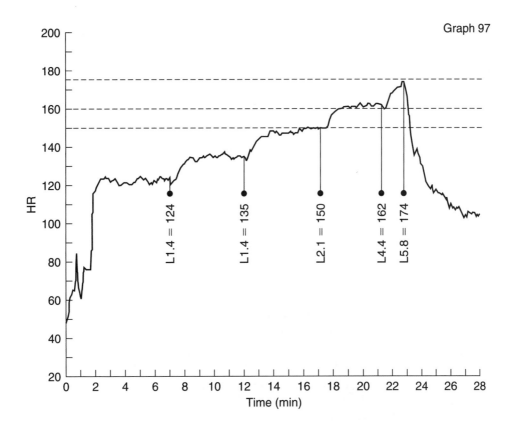

Graph 97

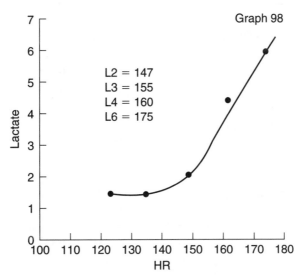

Graph 98

The MLSS is the highest constant power that an athlete can generate during 1 to 1.5 hours without lactate accumulation in the blood. The MLSS can be determined accurately on a bicycle ergometer. The cyclist can cycle for

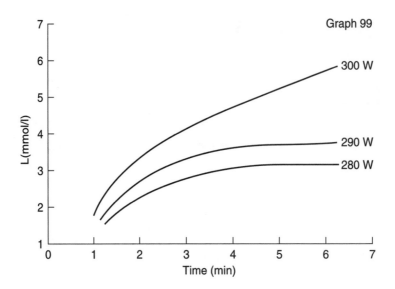

half an hour on separate days at a given wattage. On every subsequent day, the wattage is increased. During this effort, the cyclist's lactate content can be determined every 2 to 3 minutes. Lactate content will rise to a given level in the first 10 minutes and then remain constant. If the workload becomes too high, this stabilization cannot take place, and lactate content increases. The highest wattage at which lactate content remains constant is called the MLSS. The corresponding HR may be used as a training guideline.

Runners can make a sport-specific determination of the MLSS. In principle, this test is the same as the one for cyclists, that is, doing units of exercise that increase in intensity. Divide the test in units of 10 minutes. The pace is increased every 10 minutes so that the HR settles at a level 5 to 10 beats higher than the previous unit. The unit that cannot be maintained any more is too intensive. The last unit that can be run without any problem indicates the MLSS.

Another way for runners to determine MLSS is to perform an uninterrupted test, choosing a pace that can be maintained for about 1 hour. There is no intermediate or final sprint. The constant pace and the HR attained indicate the MLSS.

Endurance athletes can work toward each racing season with these basic principles for establishing the most effective training plan. These principles apply to all types of sports. First, the athlete needs to rest sufficiently (a few weeks) after the previous season. During this time the athlete should train little and can try other types of recreational sports to keep in condition. In this period a lot of endurance athletes practice some power training, because the racing season leaves little time for that. Following are descriptions of the phases of a training season.

Phase 1

This phase lasts 6 to 8 weeks, depending on the athlete's experience. After 6 to 8 weeks the body should have adapted to the new circumstances and will not adapt any further. The goal during in this period is to train basic endurance capacity, which is best achieved by doing a lot of workouts in the aerobic 1 (A1) zone; some 70% of all mileage should be in that zone. The other 30% can be divided over the other zones such as aerobic 2 (A2), endurance 1 (E1), and endurance 2 (E2).

Phase 2

The second phase also lasts 6 to 8 weeks. Now that the athlete's basic endurance capacity is well established, he or she can start training much more in the A2 zone, up to 40%, which will bring about specific adaptations. The athlete can do a limited amount of training in the higher intensity zones, E1 and E2. At this point training is sport specific; that is, the runner adapts to running and the cyclist adapts to cycling.

Phase 3

The third phase starts with high-intensity workouts in the form of either intervals or uninterrupted work. Again, the period lasts some 6 to 8 weeks. The intensity zones as percentages of the HR at the MLSS are as follows:

A1, the long, quiet endurance workouts: HR 75% to 85% of the HR at MLSS

A2, the intermediate or normal endurance workouts: HR 85% to 95% of the HR at MLSS

E1, intensive endurance or threshold training: HR 95% to 100% of the HR at MLSS

E2, high-intensity speed endurance

On the Road

The anaerobic threshold may be determined during normal exercise. This is an advantage, because the test will be sport specific. For example, when a marathon runner is tested on a bicycle ergometer, the data of the test cannot be used to assess his or her running workouts.

This is an example of lactate determination in a marathon runner where the conditions are sport specific. Lactate is determined while the athlete is running on the road, four segments of 1 kilometer with a recovery pause between each. Every successive kilometer is run faster, and a blood sample is taken after every kilometer. Above the line of the curve are the HR and corresponding lactate concentration (see graph 100).

Graph 101 indicates the following: L2 = 132, L2.5 = 135, L3 = 138, L4 = 142, and L6 = 147.

Table 4.3 and graph 102 provide another example of anaerobic threshold determination during exercise on the road. After an extensive warm-up, the athlete runs three periods of about 10 minutes. Each period is run faster but at a level pace. After every period a blood sample is taken immediately for lactate determination. Between every period of running there is a recovery

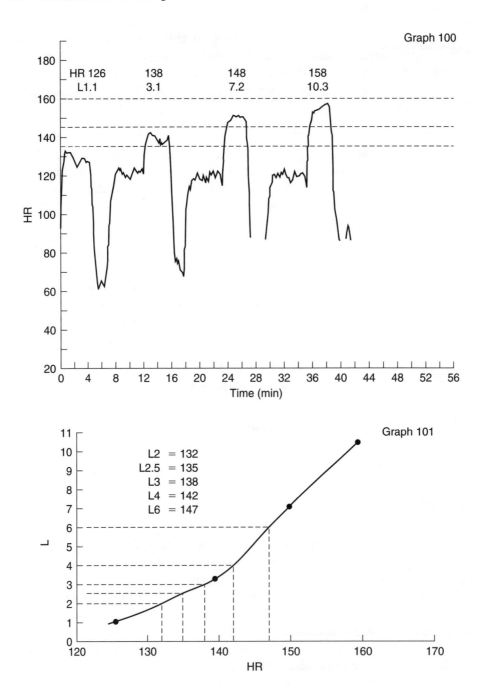

Graph 100

Graph 101

pause, which should be long enough to neutralize the lactate formed in the previous period.

These data are sufficient to construct an HR–lactate graph (graph 102). The advantage of such a determination is that the athlete is tested during a normal workout. The athlete does not lose training time, because the test itself is a good workout.

Table 4.3	Test Data	
HR		**Deduced**
HR 135 = L1.9		L2 = HR 136
HR 145 = L4.7		L3 = HR 138
HR 155 = L11.2		L4 = HR 142
		L6 = HR 147

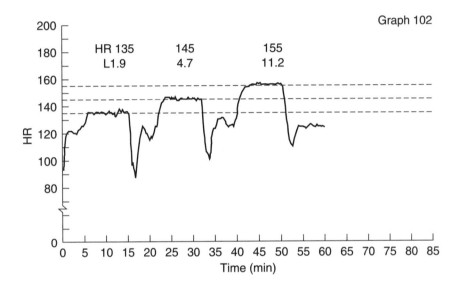

Graph 102

Practical Applications of the Lactate Test

The remainder of this chapter presents examples of applications of the lactate test. It includes advice for cyclists, runners, and other endurance athletes.

Lactate Test and Training Advice for a Cyclist

An intensive endurance workout on the road was recorded. A cyclist was told to ride maximally for 60 minutes at constant speed. The data (of even 90 minutes) show that the cyclist's HR was constantly between 160 and 165. If the intensity of the exercise was high enough, the HRdefl would be somewhere between 160 and 165. The rider cycled at maximum effort. This effort is shown in graph 103.

The data in graph 104 were obtained in a lactate test 2 days after the test on the road.

The first conclusion is that the road test, the one without lactate determination, provides a good indication of the HRdefl. The test on the road and the

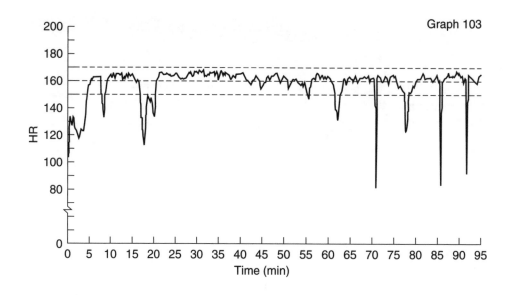

Graph 103

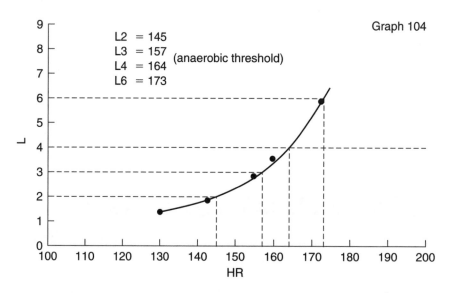

L2 = 145
L3 = 157 (anaerobic threshold)
L4 = 164
L6 = 173

Graph 104

test in the laboratory correlate very well. In both tests, the HRdefl is between 160 and 165. These data prompt the following training advice:

Recovery workouts: HR not more than 130 to 140

Extensive endurance workouts: HR between 140 and 155

Intensive endurance workouts: HR between 155 and 165

Tolerance workouts (intervals): HR more than 165

The trainer/coach and the athlete need to discuss the right mix of the total training load in relation to the race program.

Lactate Test and Training Advice for a Pro Cyclist

After a warm-up of 6 minutes, pedaling resistance is increased every 5 minutes. HR is continually measured during the test. At the end of every 5 minutes, a blood sample is taken for lactate determination (see graphs 105, and 106A, and 106B). The implications of this test are presented in table 4.4.

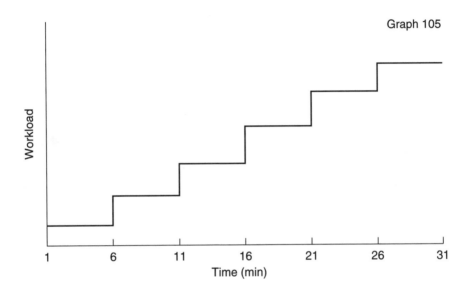

Graph 105

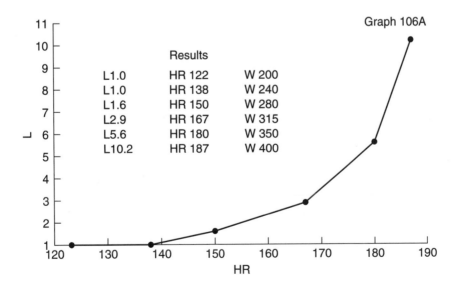

Graph 106A

Results

L1.0	HR 122	W 200
L1.0	HR 138	W 240
L1.6	HR 150	W 280
L2.9	HR 167	W 315
L5.6	HR 180	W 350
L10.2	HR 187	W 400

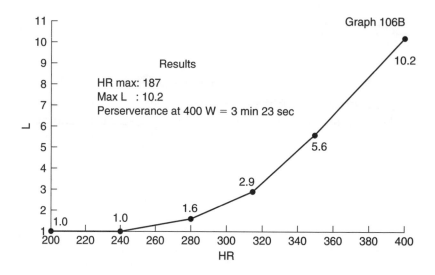

Table 4.4   Implied Values

L	HR	Power	Power/ kg body weight	% W
2.0	155 = 83% HRmax	291	3.84	72.8%
2.5	162 = 87% HRmax	304	4.01	
3.0	167 = 89% HRmax	316	4.17	
4.0	172 = 92% HRmax	329	4.34	82.3%
10.2	187 = 100% HRmax	400	5.28	

Training advice for a cyclist

Training intensities

Recovery workout: HR less than 140

This workout should be performed the day after a heavy race or workout, when the athlete has not yet completely recovered.

Training endurance capacity

Level 1: easy (A1): HR 140 to 150

Level 2: medium (A2): HR 150 to 160

Level 3: intensive (E1): HR 160 to 170

The greater part of all the cyclist's training should be endurance capacity training (about 80% to 90%).

60% at Level 1

30% at Level 2

10% at Level 3

Training lactate tolerance: HR at or more than 170

Long intervals (E2): duration 3 to 10 minutes

- Recovery: 5 to 10 minutes
- Intensity: high, HR 168 to 172
- Number of intervals: three, gradually increasing to four or five
- The cyclist should perform this workout only when well rested.

Short intervals (An1): duration 20 to 180 seconds

- Recovery: 1 to 2 minutes
- Intensity: high, HR 172 to 177
- Number of intervals: starting with five, gradually increasing to 10, 15, and 20
- The cyclist should perform this workout only when well rested.

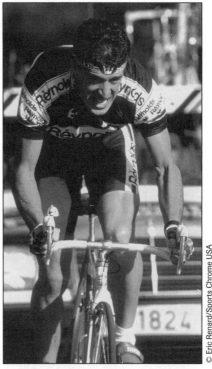

It is important for both trainer and athlete to discuss the right balance of total training load in relation to the race program.

Do not overdo lactate tolerance workouts. Once or twice a week (races included) is more than enough.

Sprint workout (An2)

Duration: short, 10 to 20 seconds

Recovery: long, 2 to 5 minutes

Intensity: high, speed far above the anaerobic threshold speed up to maximal.

Maximal HR will not be attained because of the short duration; HR will reach about 180.

Number of repetitions: starting with 3, gradually increasing to 10 to 20

Power training

Duration: long, 3 to 5 minutes

Recovery: long, 5 to 10 minutes

Intensity: moderate, from 85% to 90% maximal HR = HR 160 to 170

Number of repetitions: starting with 3, gradually increasing to 10

The cyclist should perform this workout with a heavy gear and low pedaling frequency, riding uphill or with a front wind; the cyclist should remain seated on the saddle.

Field test Form for Recording Personal Data

Lactate test

Time: afternoon

Weather conditions: dry

Place: Deurne (road)

Temperature: 16 degrees Celsius

Type of test: 3 × 10 minutes

Air humidity: high

Test leader: P.J.

Wind: none

Name: C.B.

Trainer/coach:

Birth: September 19, 1959

Sport: running 10-kilometer marathon

Particulars: none

The test results and the implications of those results are shown in graphs 107 – 109.

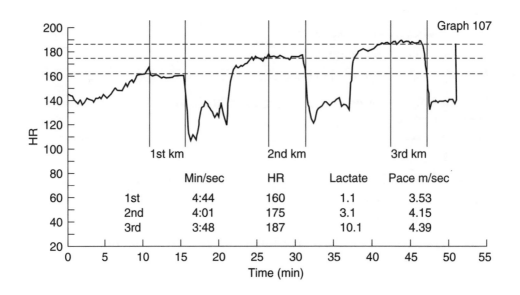

	Min/sec	HR	Lactate	Pace m/sec
1st	4:44	160	1.1	3.53
2nd	4:01	175	3.1	4.15
3rd	3:48	187	10.1	4.39

Graph 107

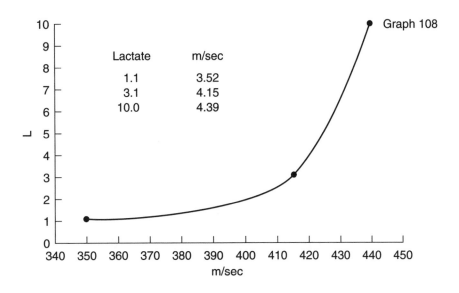

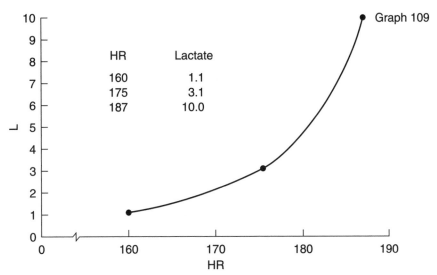

Endurance Training

For most people, aerobic endurance training should be done with lactate values between 2 and 4 millimoles per liter. Quiet, extensive endurance workouts should be between 2 and 3 millimoles per liter, and intensive endurance workouts should be between 3 and 4 millimoles per liter.

Poorly trained athletes will not always be able to avoid higher lactate values and might easily reach the following concentrations:

Intensive: 4 to 6 millimoles per liter

Extensive: 3 to 4 millimoles per liter

These athletes would be well advised to perform their workouts at a very slow pace to avoid excess acidosis. Very well trained athletes automatically train their endurance capacity at lower lactate values:

Extensive: 1.5 to 2.5 millimoles per liter

Intensive: 2.5 to 3.5 millimoles per liter

The intensity at which a marathon is run corresponds to a lactate content of 2.5 ± 0.5 millimoles per liter. The marathon time calculated for this athlete at V2.5 could be 02:56:42.

During an endurance workout, lactate content should not increase too much. If high values are reached in these workouts, tolerance will improve rather than endurance capacity. In fact, intensive workouts at high lactate values may even reduce endurance capacity. Subdivide the workout in units of 10, 15, and 20 minutes of effort, alternated by recovery periods of 5 to 10 minutes, as shown in graph 110.

Graph 110

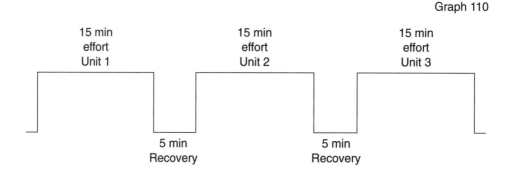

These workouts are the basis for developing and maintaining endurance capacity. Other combinations, as mentioned in the previous section, are possible, such as longer units and less recovery. If endurance capacity improves, the pace will have to be reassessed.

In tolerance training, lactate concentrations more than 4 millimoles per liter are easily reached; even values more than 10 millimoles per liter are often seen. The marathon runner should perform these workouts no more than once a week.

Two types of tolerance workouts are important for a marathon runner. The first type involves fast runs, such as a 1,000-meter run. For example, the athlete runs five segments of 1 kilometer each, at a pace faster than V4. Time should be between 00:03:45 and 00:03:55, with an HR more than 180. The runner should not take a long recovery period, not more than 2 to 3 minutes. The idea is to build up high lactate concentrations, and a recovery that is too long will decrease lactate content. The runner starts with three segments of 1 kilometer and gradually increases that to 10 segments. The number of intervals planned should be completed without time loss. If the athlete feels really worn out after three segments of 1 kilometer and the plan was to run six segments, the athlete started too fast.

The second type of tolerance workout is a run of 10 to 15 kilometers, preferably in a race, at a pace or HR just over the HRdefl, that is, just over V4 or over HR 180. In this type of race, lactate content will gradually increase to values of 6 to 10 millimoles per liter. The athlete cannot run a complete marathon at that pace, because 5 kilometers are run at 109%, 10 kilometers at 104%, and 15 kilometers at 101% of V4. The athlete should not overdo either of these workouts.

The athlete should always do a recovery workout the day after a heavy workout or race. This workout is run more slowly than V2 or below the HR at a lactate content of 2 millimoles per liter, so V2 is slower than 00:04:24 per kilometer. HR should be less than 170.

Graph 111 provides a plan for marathon training for the average runner.

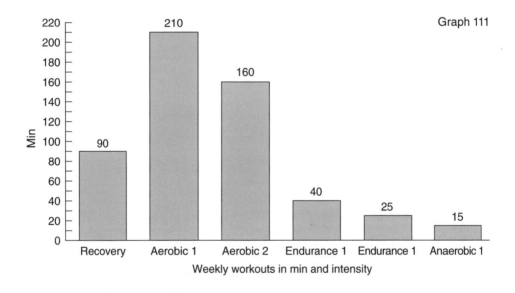

Graph 111

Summary of training

Aerobic endurance

Pace and time per kilometer	Lactate and heart rate
V2 to V4 = 00:04:24 to 00:03:54	L2 to L4 = HR 170 to 180
Extensive V2 to V3 = 00:04:24 to 00:04:00	Extensive L2 to L3, HR 170 to 175
Intensive V3 to V4 = 00:04:00 to 00:03:54	Intensive L3 to L4, HR 175 to 180

Do these workouts in units

Number of workouts: 3–4/week

Tolerance

Fast runs, for example, 1,000 meters with recovery period

1,000 meters at a pace above V4, for example, 00:03:45 to 00:03:55 per kilometer

Recovery 2 to 3 minutes

Race of about 50 minutes, for example, 15 kilometers at a pace just over V4

Coaching a Marathon Runner With the Help of HR Measurement and Lactate Determination

Name: Frits Pardoel

Age: 42

Body weight: 61.2 kilograms

Body length: 171.2 centimeters

Running history: about three marathons a year for several years

Best time: 02:40:09.

Other recent results: 02:43:00, 02:45:00, 02:58:00, 03:01:00

Maximum number of kilometers a week: about 120

On August 21, the athlete requested coaching to prepare for the Helmond Marathon on October 21. He had just recovered from an Achilles tendon injury. He ran his personal best time six years ago. Since then he was unsuccessful in every marathon. After 30 to 35 kilometers he feels worn out and his muscles are exhausted.

This athlete was advised to train in units of intensive endurance training. The HR in these units was between 140 and 145. The lactate test on the road showed that L3 and L4 corresponded with HRs of 138 and 142. The endurance workouts were deliberately set higher, because of the recent Achilles tendon injury. Once a week he ran a 15-kilometer race far above the HRdefl (HR 150 to 155). This is also seen in the lactate concentration of 9.5 millimoles per liter (see Curve 8).

This type of race trains anaerobic capacity (tolerance training). The marathon cannot be run at this intensity. The measurements show that HRs remain level. The combination of an intensive endurance workout three time per week with two recovery workouts and a tolerance workout once a week has been the ideal preparation for this athlete.

Curve 1 35-kilometer workout at marathon pace. HR is between 135 and 140 during this workout (graph 112).

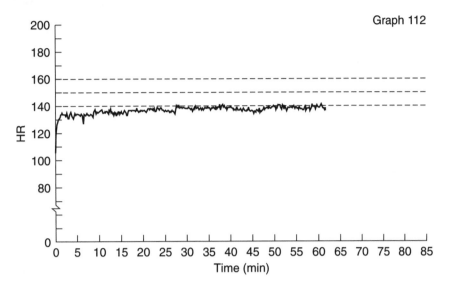

Graph 112

Curve 2 Lactate determination under sport-specific circumstances (graph 113). Lactate concentrations and corresponding HRs are as follows:

L2 at HR 132

L3 at HR 138

L4 at HR 142

L6 at HR 147

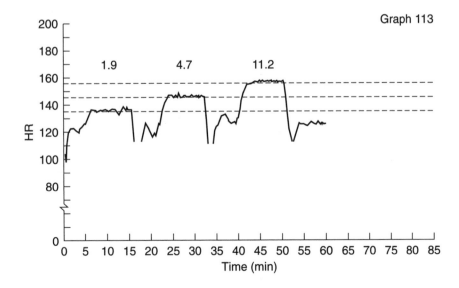

Graph 113

Curve 3 Workout with a training task. Divide the workout in units of 10 minutes. Run these units at an intensity between HR 140 and 145 (graph 114).

This workout was not effective. The athlete had not sufficiently recovered after a heavy workout the day before.

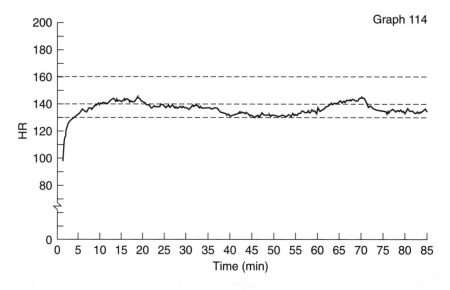

Graph 114

Curve 4 The same task as for Curve 3 but now after a day of rest (graph 115).

This workout was effective, with 41% of the workout within the correct HR range. In Curve 3, only 20% of the workout was in the right range.

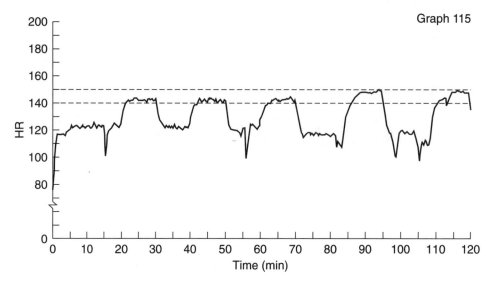

Graph 115

Curves 5–6 Workouts according to the principle of Curves 3 and 4 (graphs 116 and 117). The task was carried out perfectly.

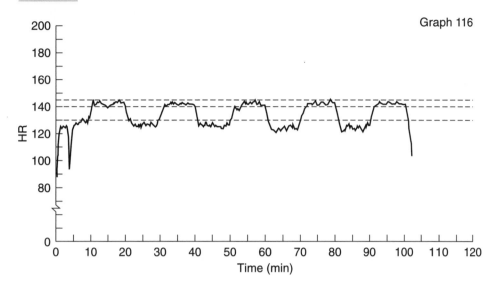

Graph 116

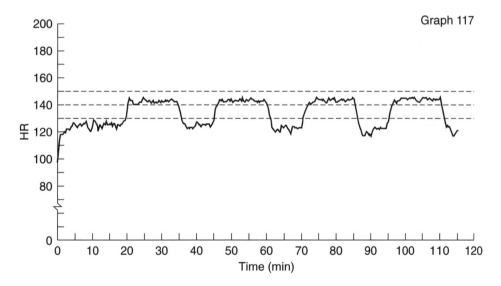

Graph 117

Curve 7 15-kilometer race; time 00:52:31; HR between 150 and 155 (graph 118).

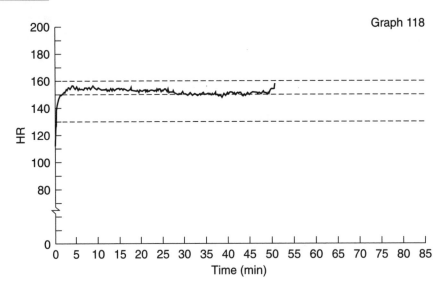

Graph 118

Curve 8 15-kilometer race; time 00:50:59 (personal best time for this distance). HR between 150 and 155. Lactate after the race 9.5 millimoles per liter (graph 119).

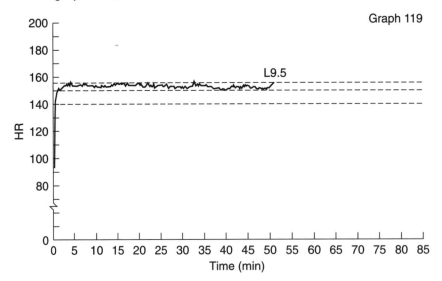

Graph 119

Curve 9 Half marathon at Venray. Task: run at an HR of about 140. Time 01:21:39 (graph 120).

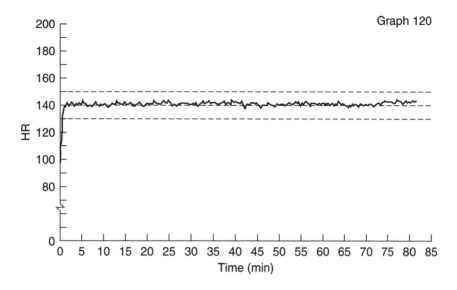

Curve 10 The Helmond marathon, run with an HR of about 140 (graph 121).

Time predicted: 02:40:00 to 02:42:00

Time actually run: 02:40:24

Best time in 6 years: average HR 141 to 142

First half of the marathon: 01:20:08

Second half of the marathon: 01:20:16

Finish: 02:40:24

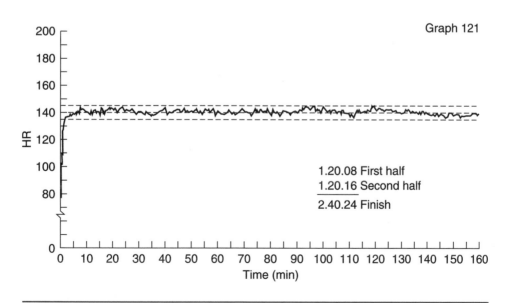

The Westland Marathon

The same runner was coached in preparation for the Westland marathon on April 12. Specific training was started in January, so the preparation time was considerably longer than for the Helmond marathon, which was in October. Because of the success of the previous preparation period, the same principle was chosen: an endurance workout three times a week, mostly in units with an HR around the HRdefl. Once a week he trained or ran a race at an intensity far above the HRdefl. The day after a heavy workout or race he trained at a very low intensity, the so-called recovery workout.

For this athlete, three endurance workouts and one tolerance workout a week were an ideal mix for an optimal preparation. In the period between October and January he trained in a very relaxed manner, with an occasional cross-country race.

Curve 11 Endurance workout of 2 hours at racing pace. Average HR between 135 and 140. On the basis of this workout, the HR for an optimal endurance workout was set at 140 to 145 (graph 122).

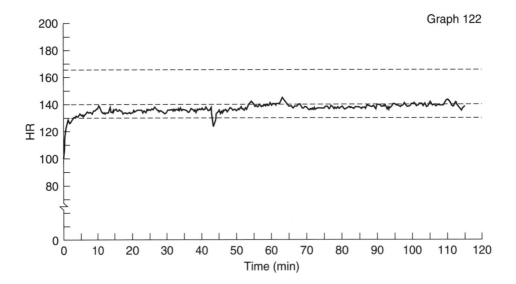

Graph 122

Curve 12

Optimal endurance workout with three units of 20 minutes, HR increasing to 145. Between the units there was a long recovery pause (graph 123).

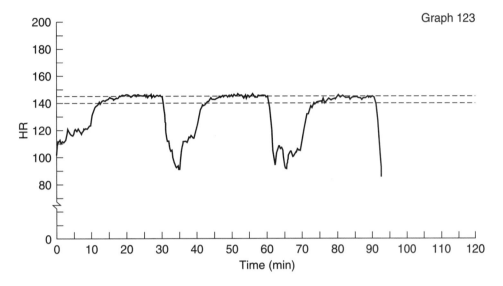

Graph 123

Curve 13

A similar workout. The units were a bit shorter, about 10 minutes (graph 124).

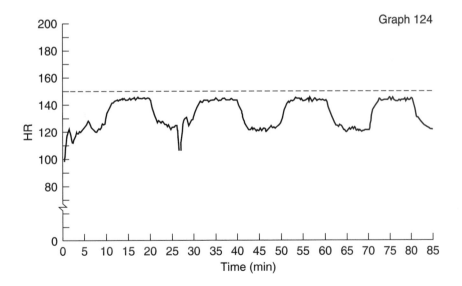

Graph 124

Curve 14
Fast run of 60 minutes. HR was constantly around 150, so above the HRdefl. This type of workout was performed once a week (graph 125).

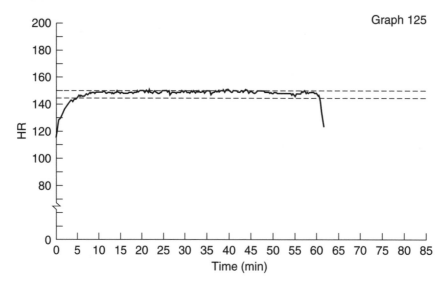

Graph 125

Curve 15
Three different units (graph 126)
Unit I: HR about 140 = extensive endurance
Unit II: HR about 145 = intensive endurance
Unit III: HR about 150 = lactate tolerance

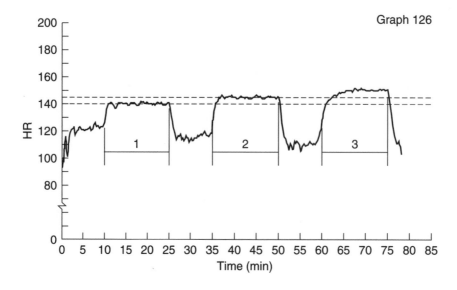

Graph 126

Curve 16

Endurance run of 60 minutes; task was set at an HR of 145. The athlete performed the run without any problem (graph 127). At about the 40th minute, the time for 1 kilometer was clocked. Time for 1 kilometer at HR 145 = 00:03:45. Calculated marathon time = 02:37:00.

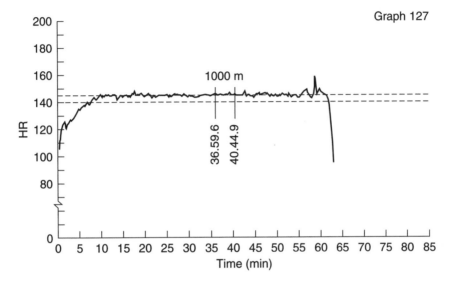

Graph 127

Curve 17

Half marathon Overloon (February 2). Cold, about 0 degrees Celsius (32 degrees Fahrenheit). Lactate content at the end of the race was 4.2 millimoles per liter. This curve shows that the athlete started too vigorously. HR at the beginning was 155 (his L4 is HR 142, see Curve 2). Gradual decrease of HR during the race. HR at the end 145. Time for half marathon: 01:21:22 (graph 128).

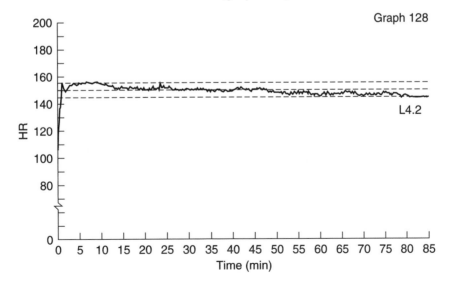

Graph 128

Curve 18   Lactate on the road during a sport-specific test.

Task: 15 minutes running at HR 140, then a long recovery pause and 15 minutes at HR 150.

After running 15 minutes with an HR of 140, lactate content is 2.8 millimoles per liter.

After running 15 minutes with an HR of 150, lactate content is 4.3 millimoles per liter.

The following values could be calculated:

L2 = HR 135

L3 = HR 142

L4 = HR 147 to 148 (graphic 129)

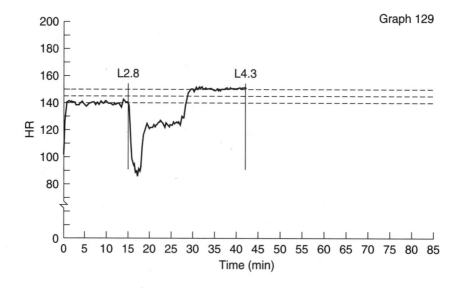

Graph 129

Compared with the Helmond marathon, the HRdefl has shifted from HR 142 to HR 147 to 148. This higher HR can be explained by a better tolerance, or possibly the athlete had rested better before the start.

| **Curve 19** | Westland marathon on April 12. Weather conditions: cold, 4 to 5 degrees Celsius (41 degrees Fahrenheit), much wind. Task: run the marathon at a pace corresponding to HR 145 (graphic 130) |

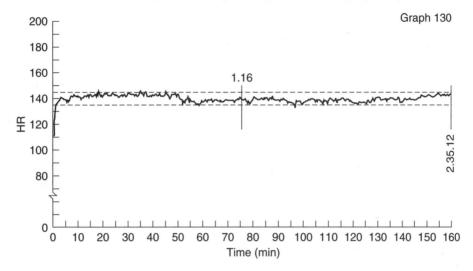

During the race, the athlete runs the first 50 minutes at HR 145. Then he joins a group of about 25 runners. Because the expected finish time is far below plan (the aim is to finish in 02:37:00), the coach, who accompanies him on a bike, advises him to stick to that group. In the shelter of this group, HR decreases distinctly. This indicates how important the role of a pacing device may be.

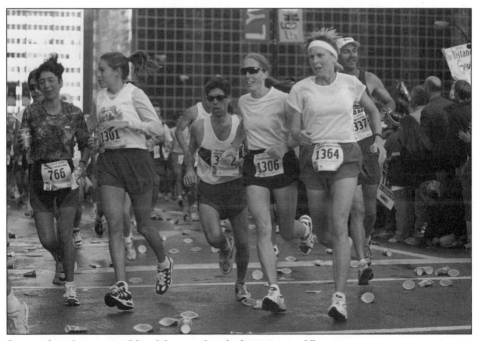

A marathon is run at a blood-lactate level of ± 2.5 mmol/l.

The first half of the marathon is covered in 01:16:00, the second half in 01:19:12. The runner finishes in 02:35:12. The athlete has had no problem at all; he felt that he could have kept up the pace of the first 50 minutes quite easily. The finish time is an improvement of his personal best time by more than 5 minutes. After the marathon the athlete has a rapid and good recovery. Progression might still be possible. A time of about 02:30:00 seems a reasonable expectation.

Field Test and Training Advice for Two Marathon Runners

The right-hand curve of graph 131 is the lactate curve of international-level marathon runners. They ran an optimal marathon at an intensity corresponding to a lactate concentration of 2.5 ± 0.5 millimoles per liter. If this marathon intensity is set at 100%, the other intensities may be deduced. Setting the marathon intensity at 100% is a bit confusing because up till now V4 pace has always been considered 100%. Marathon pace is about 94% of V4 pace.

The left-hand curve is the curve of medium-level trained marathon runners. Their optimal marathon intensity is at a lactate concentration of 3 ± 0.5 millimoles per liter. It is clear that the lactate curve shifts to the right when the level is improved.

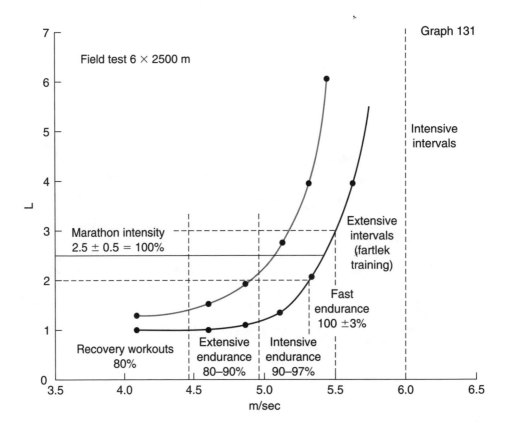

Testing and Training With Gelindo Bordin

This section contains a number of tests to check the condition of Gelindo Bordin (Olympic champion in 1988 and European marathon champion in 1990) done by Daniele Faraggiana, sports physician in Italy.

The tests were part of the training workouts, so they could be done very frequently. Every two weeks Bordin was tested on the track or a marked route. To reach a good steady-state level, test runs of 2,000 meters were chosen. The total test consisted of five to six test runs, each of 2,000 meters, which were covered at increasing pace. The choice of running paces was based on the expected pace in the marathon. The training paces were just under, equal to, and just over marathon pace.

Bordin used a pacing device, an apparatus that issues a sound signal at every 12.5 meters, which enables the runners to maintain a constant pace. During the test an HR monitor was used to measure HR. After every 2,000 meters there was a 40-second pause, during which a blood sample was taken for lactate determination (see table 4.5 and graph 132).

Table 4.5 Stepwise Test Series for Gelindo Bordin's Most Important Marathons

40-sec pause   Lactate values mmol/l–HR/ bpm

2,000-m time (min:sec)	6/12/87 L	6/12/87 HR	7/2/87 L	7/2/87 HR	8/17/87 L	8/17/87 HR	3/29/88 L	3/29/88 HR	9/16/88 L	9/16/88 HR	4/1/90 L	4/1/90 HR	8/15/90 L	8/15/90 HR
6:20	2.4	171	1.8	167	1.6	167	1.5	158						
6:15	3.0	175	2.6	171	1.9	168	1.8	161	1.9	160				
6:10	3.6	177	2.9	175	2.5	172	2.1	164	2.0	164	2.1	168		
6:05	4.3	178	3.6	179	2.6	174	2.6	170	2.2	168				
6:00	6.4	185	5.4	181	3.5	177	2.8	172	2.9	172	2.8	172	2.8	172
5:55														
5:50									3.8	173				

Race-specific endurance capacity will be improved when the lactate curve shifts to the right. The pace at 2.5 millimoles per liter has great value for predicting the athlete's marathon time and also is an important indicator for assessing pace in various types of workout. Experience has shown that a marathon runner should not run faster than the pace corresponding with a lactate value of 2.5 ± 0.5 millimoles per liter. This knowledge is psychologically important for the marathon runner, because it will make the runner more conscious of his or her possibilities and limitations.

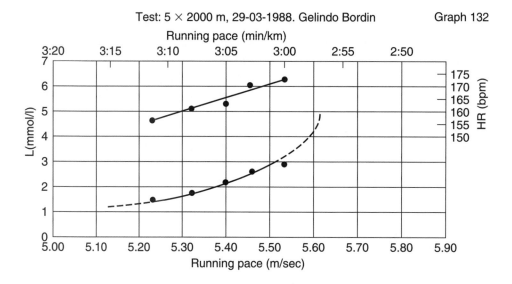

Test: 5 × 2000 m, 29-03-1988. Gelindo Bordin   Graph 132

HR is a good parameter for managing and checking the intensity of various types of workouts. With the help of an HR monitor, workouts can be conducted at certain HRs. By storing this workout HR in the memory bank of the HR monitor, the athlete or coach can check the training task afterward.

On the basis of the lactate curve (see graph 132), the athlete and coach can discuss the program of workouts and races. If the curve should shift to left or right, training intensities should be readjusted.

Marathon Training of Gelindo Bordin by Professor Luciano Gigliotti from Italy

The starting point is a marathon pace of 00:03:01 per kilometer. With this pace the marathon will be run in 02:07:16. The training volume per week is 280 kilometers.

To improve aerobic capacity, fast endurance workouts of 12 to 16 kilometers are run at 00:02:56 per kilometer and interval workouts of 3 × 7 kilometers. The first 7 kilometers are run in 00:02:59, the second 7 in 00:02:58, and the last 7 in 00:02:55. Between the 7-kilometer sections, there is a pause of 1 kilometer in 00:03:10. This means that the fast runs and intervals are run at a pace faster than marathon pace of 00:03:01 per kilometer. The intensities, just over or just under marathon pace, differ 2.5 seconds per 1,000 meters.

The lactate range within which aerobic capacity will be trained is between 2.5 and 3.5 millimoles per liter. Gigliotti does not believe marathon runners should perform workouts in which high lactate values are reached. These high lactate values are not considered suitable for efficient marathon training.

A cycle targeted at training volume is subdivided as follows:

85% of all the training work under 2 millimoles per liter

10% of all the training work between 2 and 4 millimoles per liter

5% of all the training work above 4 millimoles per liter

A cycle targeted at high intensity is subdivided as follows:

75% of all the work under 2 millimoles per liter

15% between 2 and 4 millimoles per liter

5% above 4 millimoles per liter

Bordin runs his long endurance workouts relatively fast. In a workout of 02:30:00, the first hour is run at 00:03:30 per kilometer; the second hour at 00:03:20 per kilometer, and the last 30 minutes at 00:03:10 per kilometer. The total running distance of such a workout is nearly 46 kilometers. Gigliotti is opposed to the idea of long, slow distance training.

Due to sensitive Achilles tendons, Bordin does not train on the athletics track. He does his short intervals on the road in the form of minute-runs such as 10 × 1.5 minutes with a 1.5-minute pause or 10 × 1 minute with a 1-minute pause.

Table 4.6 shows the last period of specific marathon training by Gelindo Bordin. This specific period of 12 to 13 weeks is subdivided into four cycles.

During the altitude workouts (2,400 meters), the intensity of endurance runs is adjusted downward, from 00:02:58 to 00:03:08 per kilometer. The altitude stage is finished 2.5 weeks before the marathon. The table shows that there is another, earlier, altitude stage in this specific marathon training period. During these two altitude stages, the emphasis lies on increasing training volume. Back at sea level, the emphasis lies on intensity again, except for the last week.

Table 4.6 Gelindo Bordin's Training Program of June to August 1991

Period	Training targets	km/week	Particulars
1. 3-4 weeks	First increase of training volume, improvement of aerobic capacity	240-260	Altitude training
2. 3 weeks	Improvement of race specific endurance	220-240	Sea level, fewer higher intensities
3. 3.5 weeks	Second increase of training volume, improvement of aerobic capacity and specific endurance	260-280	Altitude training
4. 2.5 weeks	Attaining top condition	220-260	Sea level except last week

Improving the Marathon With the Help of HR Measurement

This section compares two marathons. The first is the Eindhoven marathon, October 1986, and the second is the Helmond marathon, October 1987.

In the Eindhoven marathon (graph 133), from the start to the 25th kilometer, HR is above 165. So this runner can keep performing over his HRdefl for 1 hour and 50 minutes. Then he cannot keep up the pace any more and is forced to slow down. His HR decreases as well. His first 20 kilometers are covered in 01:23:27 and the second 20 kilometers in 01:54:42. Total marathon time is 03:27:28.

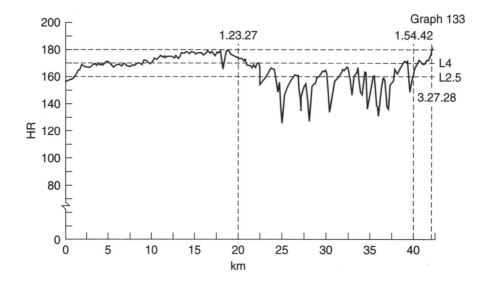

This is a classic example of a marathon failure. After a few tests, training intensities are adjusted (test April) and the right marathon pace is set (test September).

The test data in table 4.7 show that the HR levels have not changed very much between April and September. On the other hand, performance level has increased enormously. The calculated marathon time at a lactate content of 2.5 millimoles per liter (V2.5) has improved from 03:09:00 to 02:53:00 (see graph 134).

In the Helmond marathon in October 1987, the athlete made a prudent start, keeping his HR under 160 at the beginning. Later in the race, HR was between 160 and 165. From 2 hours onward, HR was between 165 and 170.

This was a personal best time, for the first time within 3 hours. At the beginning of the marathon the runner kept the pace low deliberately. This marathon was built up well and run at level pace.

Table 4.7   Test Data

April 1987	September 1987
L 2 = HR 155	L 2 = HR 156
L 3 = HR 160	L 3 = HR 161
L 4 = HR 165	L 4 = HR 165
V2 = 3.64 m/sec	V2 = 4.00 m/sec
V3 = 3.78 m/sec	V3 = 4.10 m/sec
V4 = 3.95 m/sec	V4 = 4.19 m/sec
V2.5 = 03:09:00	V2.5 = 02:53:00

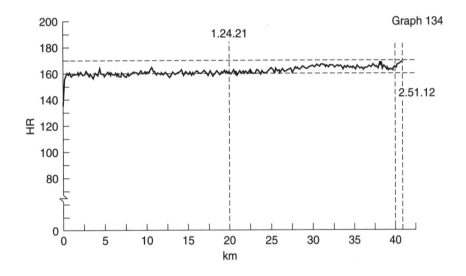

Graph 134

Example of Training Advice for a Female Swimmer

Female: 14 years old

Sport: Swimming

Category: Competition

Union: KNZB

Name: Van der AA

First name: Ellen

Place: swimming pool, Gemert test 4 × 300-meter freestyle

Place: Gemert

Time: evening

Particulars: No further development in the last 18 months, despite many intensive workouts. Workouts probably have been too intensive

Target: Adjusting the right training intensities.

Best times: 1985: 100 meters 00:01:02.3, 200 meters 00:02:15.9, 400 meters 00:04:38 1986: 100 meters 00:01:05.5, 200 meters 00:02:18

Test:

10 minutes warm-up	time	m/sec	m/min	L
300 meters, pause 5 minutes	00:05:01	0.99	59.80	1.7
300 meters, pause 5 minutes	00:04:01	1.24	74.68	5.2
300 meters, pause 10 minutes	00:03:48	1.32	78.95	8.4
300 meters, pause 10 minutes	00:03:40	1.36	81.81	9.6
100 meters	00:01:05	1.54	93.31	13.9

Implied values

L2 = 1.16 meters per second = V2
L3 = 1.18 meters per second = V3
L4 = 1.21 meters per second = V4
L5 = 1.23 meters per second = V5
L6 = 1.27 meters per second = V6

The test was excellent. Three measuring points above L4 are in one line. V4 is 1.21 meters per second. On the German national level, V4 is between 1.20 and 1.30 meters per second. On the European level, V4 is between 1.40 and 1.50 meters per second. On worldwide and Olympic levels, V4 is between 1.50 and 1.87 meters per second. During the test, the swimmer reached levels above L4 rather fast. After the second 300 meters, lactate content had already increased to 5.2 millimoles per liter. This confirms the idea that training intensities have been too high in the past.

Training advice

Swim 400 meters at V4 speed a number of times.

The 400 meters will be in 00:05:31.

The swimmer should get to know what it feels like to swim at L4.

The swimmer should have her split times checked and written down. In that way she can check whether she swims at a constant speed.

400-meter times should constantly be between 00:05:26 and 00:05:34.

The swimmer should perform recovery workouts at L2 or even less intensively.

1. Do not race or perform intensive tolerance workouts more often than once a week. These workouts have very high lactate concentrations, up to 8 and higher. In the 100-meter sprint, the swimmer reaches a lactate content of 13.9. The swimmer should always perform a recovery workout the day after a race or a workout that turned out to be very heavy.

2. She should train her endurance capacity at L2, L3, L4, and L5.

3. She should perform the following sprint workouts.

    a. Five to 10 100-meter sprints, with a 30- to 45-second pause, preferably with quiet swimming during the pause. Perform the sprints without diving. Swimming speed = 1.29 meters per second, so 100 meters in 00:01:17 or 00:01:18.

    b. Ten to 15 50-meter sprints with a 30- to 45-second pause. Swimming speed = 1.43 meters per second, so 50 meters in about 35 seconds.

    c. Ten to 20 25-meter sprints with a 30- to 45-second pause. Swimming speed = 1.57 meters per second, so 25 meters in 15 to 16 seconds (see table 4.8).

Training based on the preceding program improved the swimmer's performance in the first 6 weeks. Her plateau in performance of the last 18 months was broken remarkably soon. The times of the 100-meter freestyle illustrated that 100-meter times in the last 18 months were always around 00:01:05, mostly a little bit more than that. Her 100-meter times in the last six weeks were 00:01:03.8, 00:01:03, 00:01:02.6, and 00:01:02.2. Her personal best time for this distance improved, and the other distances were improved considerably.

Table 4.8 Endurance Workouts

		V4 = 1.21 m/sec			
		Extensive (min:sec)		**Intensive (min:sec)**	
Number•	**Pause (sec)**	**L2**	**L3**	**L4**	**L5**
100 m	10	1:23	1:21	1:19	1:18
	30	1:20	1:19	1:17	1:15
200 m	10	2:47	2:45	2:40	2:38
	30	2:45	2:42	2:38	2:36
400 m	10	5:38	5:32	5:24	5:19
	30	5:36	5:29	5:21	5:15
		Average time per 100 m			
20-45 min of endurance training		1:27	1:25	1:23	1:21

*Number of repetitions at least 3 to 4×.

chapter 5

Overtraining

The athlete achieves better performance through training. Training disturbs a certain equilibrium within the body, and recovery after training is necessary to find a new equilibrium.

Supercompensation

If the volume and intensity of the workout are correct and the resting period is long enough, the body not only recovers but exceeds its previous capacity. We call this the *supercompensation period*. Graphs 135 and 136 illustrate the principle of supercompensation.

Recovery is an essential part of training. All too often athletes train with the notion "the more, the better," and they neglect sufficient rest and recovery. The danger of overtraining is very great then, because without a recovery period, there will be no supercompensation and training cannot be effective. However, if the recovery period is too long, the benefits of supercompensation will not last. So training well is an art, and it requires finding the right balance between workloads and recovery periods.

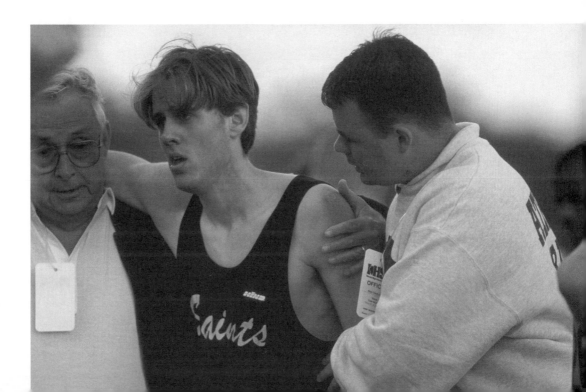

Graph 135

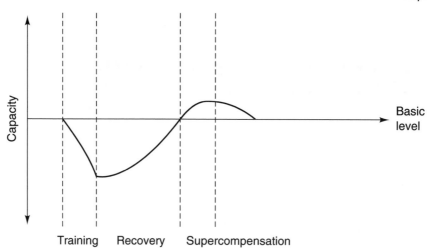

Training   Recovery   Supercompensation

Graph 136

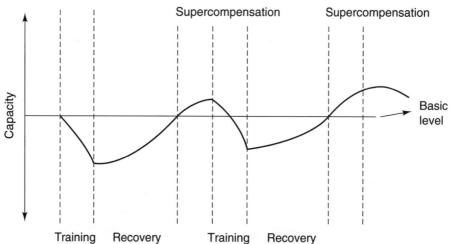

Training   Recovery   Training   Recovery

This is complicated by the fact that recovery time is not a constant factor but rather differs among training methods. The length of this recovery period depends on the following:

- Method of training
- Athlete's training experience
- Degree of exhaustion

- Athlete's age
- Athlete's physical ability to recover

The supercompensation model explains why athletes who train too much and take inadequate recovery periods become overloaded (see graph 137). This practice inevitably and cumulatively decreases the athlete's basic level of capacity. In the long run, overtraining will result.

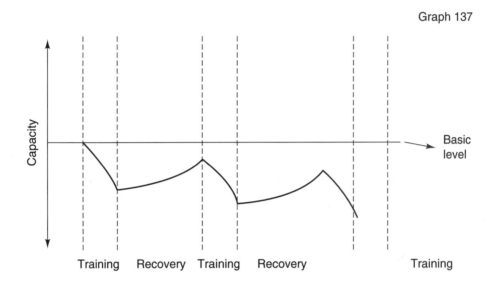

The hormonal system and the nervous system both play an important role in recovery. The hormonal and the nervous system work together but are directed and coordinated in a center in the brain. The main task of this center, the hypothalamus, is to enable the body to react adequately to difficult circumstances. Those circumstances may be physical exercise, such as a heavy workout, but also psychological stress such as problems at home or at work. The hypothalamus can handle a certain amount of physical and psychological stress. However, if the critical limit is surpassed, the hormonal and nervous systems become disordered, which is exactly what happens in overtraining. Attendant circumstances that play an important role include the following:

- Personal problems (private or job related)
- Examination period at school
- Too many races
- Fear of failure
- Nutritional deficiencies

- Change of climate
- Jet lag
- Infectious diseases
- Allergic reactions
- Altitude training

These circumstances temporarily reduce the body's capability to carry loads. If an athlete ignores these factors and continues to train hard, despite diminished capability, he or she will fall into a downward spiral, which will eventually result in overtraining.

Many athletes tend to train too much and too intensively, which will increase exhaustion and decrease performance level. If timely and sufficient rest is taken, a complete recovery might be possible within a few days. Many athletes, however, interpret this faster exhaustion as a signal of insufficient training, and heighten their training load. Then they overstress the nervous and hormonal systems, and symptoms of the overtraining syndrome will result. The first symptoms of overtraining are hyperactivity of the sympathetic nervous system.

Symptoms of Sympathetic Overtraining

One or more of the following symptoms may be seen in the case of sympathetic overtraining:

- Poor recovery of heart rate (HR) after exercise
- Higher HR at rest
- Exhaustion occurring sooner
- Decreased appetite and weight loss
- Heart palpitations
- Poor sports performance
- More sore muscles
- Increased risk of injuries
- Increased risk of infections
- Emotional instability
- Troubled sleep
- Nervousness
- Irritability
- Loss of concentration
- Feeling of agitation
- Increased perspiration
- Decreased enthusiasm for training

At the first symptoms of sympathetic overtraining, workouts should be decreased drastically and immediately. If the right measures are taken quickly, improvement can be reached in a few weeks. This type of overtraining is seen often in athletes who train very intensively. The highly intensive interval workouts, performed too often, are especially notorious for leading to sympathetic overtraining. These workouts require a recovery period of about 3 days. The number of intensive interval workouts, races included, should not be more than two per week.

If the athlete neglects the symptoms of sympathetic overtraining and continues to train excessively, the hormonal and nervous systems become exhausted. The parasympathetic nervous system then becomes dominant. This type of overtraining is called parasympathetic overtraining, and its symptoms are opposite those of sympathetic overtraining.

Symptoms of Parasympathetic Overtraining

Some symptoms of parasympathetic overtraining are as follows:

- Body weight constant and appetite normal
- Often a normal recovery of HR after exercise
- Lower HR at rest
- Poor performance
- Depression
- Fatigue
- Sleepiness
- Lethargy
- Low blood pressure
- Hypoglycemia
- More enthusiasm for training

Parasympathetic overtraining is often seen in endurance athletes who train with a large training volume. Recovery from parasympathetic overtraining may take weeks or even months.

How to Recognize Overtraining

Although thorough questioning may lead to the diagnosis of overtraining, a major factor is an athlete's poor performance. Determining the lactate curve may provide important information as well. In these cases, it is important to compare the test data with tests from periods when the athlete was not overtrained. In cases of overtraining, the athlete will have lower lactate values at maximal or submaximal effort, which is called the lactate paradox.

The Lactate Paradox

As condition improves, the lactate curve will shift to the right. But under certain circumstances, a rightward shift does not indicate an improvement, which causes some problems in interpreting the lactate curve (see graph 138).

Carbohydrates are needed for the formation of lactate, and when carbohydrate depots are not full, the formation of lactate is disturbed and different lactate curves may result. Situations in which carbohydrate depots are not sufficiently filled include the day after an exhausting workout, fatigue, periods of fasting, long endurance exercise, and all forms of overtraining. In those cases, glycolysis is disturbed and lactate content during exercise will remain low.

In cases of insufficiently filled carbohydrate depots or in cases of overtraining, lactate values, for both light and strenuous exercise, are paradoxically low. With such a lactate paradox, condition may seem to be improved, but exactly the opposite is true. With a lactate paradox, the HR–lactate curve shifts to the right. This shift is accompanied by diminished maximal capacity, and in most cases maximal lactate values and maximal HR are not reached.

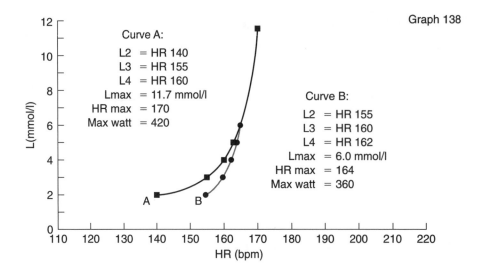

Graph 138

Curve A:

L2 = HR 140
L3 = HR 155
L4 = HR 160
Lmax = 11.7 mmol/l
HR max = 170
Max watt = 420

Curve B:

L2 = HR 155
L3 = HR 160
L4 = HR 162
Lmax = 6.0 mmol/l
HR max = 164
Max watt = 360

To achieve a valid lactate curve, the athlete must meet certain demands. Only when lactate testing is performed under equal circumstances can results be compared and the correct conclusions drawn.

It is important to know what speed or what power is reached at maximal lactate content. For top athletes in good condition, the combination of high maximum speed and relatively low lactate content is very well possible. A lactate level of L3.5 accompanied by a speed of 50 kilometers per hour is no lactate paradox but rather top condition.

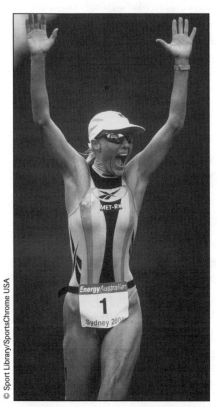

Combining high speed and low lactate helps Michellie Jones take home the 2000 Sydney Triathlon World Cup.

The HR Monitor and Overtraining

A slight increase in resting HR of four to five beats may indicate an incomplete recovery. Thus, overtraining may be traced at an early stage by measuring the morning pulse. Measuring HR during the night provides even more information about possible overtraining. During endurance exercise, the athlete will notice that keeping up a normal training pace is more difficult and results in a higher HR. In case of the sympathetic form of overtraining, the HR may decrease less rapidly after exercise.

The HR monitor may be an adequate aid for building up a training program and checking intensities, so that excessive loads may be avoided. It is necessary, however, to investigate all other possible causes for overtraining symptoms. Some of these are anemia; infectious diseases, especially viral diseases such as mononucleosis and influenza; disorders of the thyroid gland, kidneys, or adrenal glands; disorders of the heart muscle; and diabetes. These causes can only be excluded after an extensive medical investigation.

A training diary may be a tremendous aid for the early recognition of the symptoms of overtraining. Diary entries that indicate a heightened morning pulse, changes in body weight, and poorer training times, despite an equal or increased volume and/or intensity, should prompt evaluation of the training program.

Causes of Overtraining

There are many causes of overtraining, including the training process itself, races, the athlete's lifestyle, social surroundings, and health.

Errors in the Training Process

There is potential for many kinds of errors in training. Workloads can be increased too fast, or the athlete might observe insufficient recovery after exercise. The intensities may be too high for extensive endurance training, and the volume may be too high for intensive interval workouts. The athlete who trains too soon and too intensively after an illness or injury risks overtraining. Any inflexible rule in the training program can be dangerous. Whether a day of rest is necessary depends on many factors.

Races

Too many races in a short period of time can lead to overtraining. Poor sleep before an event coupled with a faulty training program can also cause problems. The fear of failure and extreme pressure from sponsors, media, or relatives cause some athletes to overtrain.

Lifestyle

An athlete's lifestyle can lead to overtraining. An irregular way of living (e.g., working on a night shift), insufficient sleep, and no recreational activities contribute to the problem. Of course, smoking and alcohol abuse are detrimental to a training program.

Social Surroundings

The athlete's social life influences his or her training. Tensions with family and friends are stressful. An athlete who is overloaded at work or school is at risk for overtraining symptoms, and being unhappy with school or a job also can be detrimental.

Health

Infectious diseases are bound to affect training. Chronic inflammations, such as tonsillitis, laryngitis, or sinusitis, also will weaken defenses. The athlete with disordered digestion, fever, anemia, or diarrhea cannot expect to train with the usual intensity. Even dental problems will affect training.

Some Specific Health Problems

Some health problems occur in athletes so often that they warrant discussion here. They are viral infections, one type of which is mononucleosis.

Viral Infections

Viral infections are very common. One adult may go through six viral infections a year. The most common viruses in humans are the influenza virus (which causes the flu), the rhinovirus (which causes colds), the Coxsackievirus, the adenovirus, the cytomegalovirus, and the Epstein-Barr virus (which is responsible for mononucleosis, as discussed in the next section). Viral infections are mostly situated in the throat and bronchial tubes. The virus penetrates the cell and multiplies there, after which the cell breaks and new viruses are released. Viral infections may be asymptomatic, but the patient may also have many complaints, such as fatigue, rapid exhaustion after physical exercise, and sore muscles. Antibiotics do not affect viruses. Most viral infections are minor; the person does not feel fit for a few days, but everyday life can go on as usual. However, the seriousness of the disease may vary widely, and the course of the infection is determined in large part by the body's resistance.

Athletes training intensively are more susceptible to diseases than nonathletes. Athletes are more exposed to inclement weather, especially cyclists, who are notorious for their bronchial infections during workouts early in the season. Moreover, athletes are often members of large groups and may have more exposure to viruses. Intensive workouts temporarily undermine athletes' immune systems, making them more susceptible to viral infections.

Viral infections can damage muscle tissue, including the heart muscle. Sudden heart death during intensive exercise may be a complication of a viral infection. Some of the viruses mentioned here, especially the Coxsackie virus, can cause an inflammation of the heart muscle (myocarditis), which may cause sudden death during exercise. During viral infections, training should never be intensive and when a fever is present, training should be stopped temporarily. Asthmatic athletes should be very careful during bronchial infections, because exercise may evoke an asthmatic attack.

The athlete performs poorly when ill with a virus; he or she can handle workloads less easily and may soon experience overtraining if training intensity is not adjusted. Viral infections influence sports performance through malfunctioning of the ventilatory track and the heart. In addition, muscular strength may diminish by 15% during viral infections. Thus, mild viral infections may be the cause of an unexplained loss of condition. When loss of condition cannot otherwise be explained, a medical check-up to exclude a viral infection is called for.

It is difficult to determine when the athlete can resume training after a viral infection. Mild infections require a temporary decrease of intensity, but in cases of serious and long-lasting complaints, such as mononucleosis (see following section), the program should be stopped completely and resumed only when the symptoms have fully disappeared. Then the training program should be resumed gradually, starting with endurance workouts in which HRs do not surpass 140.

In the last few years, scientists have come to know more about the relationships among exercise, infections, and immunity. Although there is still much to investigate, there are some common opinions.

The most important finding is that exercise, infections, and immunity are related. Moderate forms of endurance training stimulate the immune system. Long-lasting and exhausting forms of exercise suppress the immune system, making the athlete more susceptible to infection. Exercise can result in tissue damage, which might act as an infectious agent. The turning point at which stimulation turns into suppression is probably about 70% of the maximum effort. Less is known about the duration of the effort. Because minerals like zinc and copper play an important role in a well-functioning immune system, supplementation for athletes undergoing long, intensive endurance workouts is recommended. Hygiene, good nutrition, sufficient rest, and vaccinations diminish the chance of infections. Administering immunoglobulins makes sense for athletes who have enhanced risk of infection.

Mononucleosis

Many athletes experience mononucleosis during their careers, and there are some persistent misconceptions about this disease. For example, some sports journalists write about this disease out of ignorance and a desire for sensation. Therefore, this section deals with the subject in detail to eliminate the many false notions and to teach the athlete how to handle infectious diseases.

Mononucleosis is known under several names. Other names for the same infection are glandular fever, Pfeiffer's disease, and "kissing" disease. The disease is caused by the Epstein-Barr virus. The symptoms typical of mononucleosis also can be caused by other viruses, such as the cytomegalia virus and the human immunodeficiency virus. To make it even more confusing, infections of the Epstein-Barr virus do not always evoke the typical symptoms of mononucleosis. For example, in young children, Epstein-Barr viral infections may cause few or no symptoms at all. On the other hand, older children and adults with this disease can be very ill indeed. In Western Europe, the peak of mononucleosis is in the age range of 15 to 25. This differs greatly from developing countries, where nearly every child has had the disease before the age of 10.

Incubation time, that is, the time between exposure to the infection and the outbreak of the disease, is 4 to 7 weeks. Contamination takes place via the saliva of the carrier, hence the name "kissing" disease. All infected persons, whether contaminated recently or a long time ago, are life long carriers; the Epstein-Barr virus, just like the herpes virus, remains present in the body for life. Although a person remains a carrier after an infection, it is not certain that the virus is constantly produced. Under certain circumstances—when resistance is low—the virus may be reactivated.

Mononucleosis has many symptoms. In 90% of the cases, the young adult experiences a sore throat, painfully swollen glands, fever, and an overall feeling of weakness. Other symptoms, occurring in various degrees, are headaches, perspiration, coughing, and sore muscles. A patient without a sore throat and painfully swollen glands is not likely to have mononucleosis. Glands in the armpits and groin may also be swollen. On examining the throat, even experienced doctors cannot distinguish between a bacterial infection and mononucleosis. Small hemorrhages on the palate are seen in 50% of the cases. One third of the patients have swollen eyelids. In 10% of the cases a light rash is seen all over the body. Half the patients have an enlarged spleen, and in 10% the liver is also swollen. Real jaundice is rare. A mild inflammation of the liver is the rule, but it never leads to lasting liver damage.

Mononucleosis may easily be confused with other disorders, including bacterial tonsillitis, cytomegalovirus infections, viral hepatitis, influenza, and AIDS. Bacterial tonsillitis results in inflammation of the throat caused by a bacterium; the swollen lymphatic glands are limited to the neck area and the feeling of general weakness is less pronounced. Cytomegalovirus infections are seldom accompanied by a sore throat; a general feeling of weakness and fever are the most striking characteristics. Viral hepatitis symptoms are jaundice, nausea, and vomiting; swollen glands and sore throat are absent. In the acute phase, influenza causes fever, fatigue, and a general feeling of weakness; like mononucleosis, influenza may cause a long-lasting fatigue. Acute AIDS infection symptoms are manifold and may look like mononucleosis.

The Diagnosis of Mononucleosis

A blood smear examined via microscope may assist in diagnosis of mononucleosis, but it cannot offer 100% certainty. The blood smear shows an increase in the number of lymphocytes, which look atypical and irritated. However, infections by the cytomegalovirus and the AIDS virus show identical blood smears. Just to make the difference between these three viruses even more complicated, all these viruses can also cause hepatitis. That means we see the same disturbed blood smears and the same liver disorders in those viral infections.

The diagnosis of mononucleosis stands when the presence of the Epstein-Barr virus can be established. This is possible because antibodies against the Epstein-Barr virus show up in the blood sometime after the infection. When these antibodies are present in the blood, the diagnosis of mononucleosis based on Epstein-Barr virus infection is 100% certain.

These antibodies, called heterophilous antibodies, are generated in the acute phase of the disease. After the acute phase they disappear again. Therefore, they cannot be used to establish an old infection and consequent immunity. These heterophilous antibodies are traced by a process called the Paul/Bunnell reaction.

It is a complicating factor that a positive Paul/Bunnell reaction occurs rather late in the acute phase of the disease. Only 50% of the cases have a positive reaction in the first week, 70% in the second week, and 90% in the third week. Thus, a negative Paul/Bunnell reaction does not exclude mononucleosis in a patient. It may be that the reaction is negative but a positive reaction is found later. The reaction remains negative in 10% of the patients with mononucleosis.

Unfortunately, these heterophilous antibodies cannot be used to mark the end of the infection. The remaining positive Paul/Bunnell reaction varies from patient to patient and it is certainly no standard for the duration and degree of illness. The Paul/Bunnell reaction is no more than a tool for diagnosing mononucleosis.

Negative Paul/Bunnell Reaction

If the Paul/Bunnell reaction remains negative after repeated tests, and thus it is impossible to prove the presence of heterophilous antibodies, one should consider another cause for the illness. However, if the suspicion of mononucleosis remains, further blood tests are available for virus-specific antibodies against the Epstein-Barr virus—the immunoglobin M and immunoglobin G antibodies. With the same blood sample, a test for immunoglobin M antibodies against the cytomegalovirus can be done. After consultation with the patient, an AIDS test might also be desirable. In that case the test should be done some weeks after the onset of the disease, because it takes some time before sufficient antibodies for a positive AIDS test are present in the blood. The acute AIDS infection, which also may show different symptoms, should not be excluded, certainly not for high-risk groups.

The Course of the Disease

It is clear that the symptoms of mononucleosis vary widely, and the course of the disease differs in every patient in both duration and degree of illness.

The fever and throat inflammation are gone in 2 weeks. The blood aspect and liver disorders also normalize again in that period. But it may take weeks or even months before the general feelings of weakness, fatigue, and exhaustion have disappeared. Therefore, mononucleosis is notorious in the world of sports. A complicating factor is that complaints caused by mononucleosis may gradually evolve into psychological complaints, and so resuming normal physical activities should not be delayed too long.

In the acute phase, the first 2 to 4 weeks, it is advisable to stop all sports activities. After this period, training usually may resume, guided by the patient's feeling of well-being. The athlete should be aware that the disease and the subsequent inactivity have undermined his or her condition, and that training must be progressed gradually. Most athletes will want to reach their former level of conditioning too quickly and will push themselves too hard, becoming entangled in a downward spiral that actually delays their progress by weeks or even months. An unbalanced buildup of training after a recent infectious disease is one of the best-known causes of overtraining.

Complications

Complications of mononucleosis are rare. The most important complication is a spleen rupture, which may even be fatal. A spleen rupture is said to occur in one out of every 1,000 cases. The rupture is caused by a slight trauma in the acute phase, that is, always in the first month of the disease. In this period, the spleen is enlarged and physical exercise should be avoided. Mononucleosis patients with painful bellies or shoulders might have a spleen rupture.

Other complications include an extrabacterial infection of the tonsils, meningitis or encephalitis, and anemia. Often, mononucleosis is misdiagnosed as a bacterial infection, and antibiotics are prescribed. In 50% of those cases there will be an allergic skin reaction. This is not only an annoying complication, but it often leads to a life-long inability to take penicillin. It is better to exclude the possibility of mononucleosis in every adolescent or young adult before antibiotics are prescribed.

Treatment

There is no special treatment for mononucleosis. The disease follows a natural course, which means that recovery will be spontaneous. Because there is nearly always a mild inflammation of the liver, the use of alcohol is not advised in the first 4 weeks after the outbreak of the disease. Physical exercise and work can be resumed based on the patient's feeling of well-being.

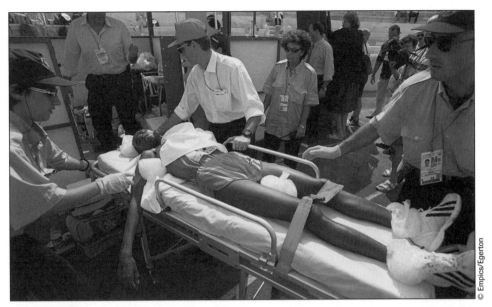

Ethiopian runner Elfenesh Alemu is rushed to an ambulance after collapsing at the finish of the women's triathlon.

Steps to be taken in case of overtraining

- Get sufficient mental rest.
- Engage in sufficient recreation.
- Take active rest in fresh air and quiet surroundings, such as walking. Passive rest is not advised, because a complete prohibition of physical activity mostly leads to more discomfort.
- Eat food rich in vitamins.
- Take extra massages, baths, and saunas.
- Do not race for a few weeks.
- Diminish training activities for 1 or 2 weeks, that is, 50% of the normal pattern in volume and intensity.
- Diminish intensity; this means no interval workouts, and intensity should not be higher than 75% of the maximum HR.
- Do all workouts with a light gear (cyclists).
- When all the symptoms have disappeared training activities can be resumed, first by gradually increasing volume and later by increasing intensity, until the normal pattern is reached.
- Only when intensive workouts can be done without problems should the athlete resume racing.

chapter 6

Circulation

The heart is a muscle pump. By contracting (which produces a heartbeat), the heart pushes blood through the arteries to the body. At rest, the heart handles an average of 4 to 5 liters of blood per minute. The blood transports oxygen and nutrients to the organs and muscles and carries waste products to the kidneys and liver.

The Heart

The heart consists of a left half and a right half, each of which consists of an atrium and a ventricle. A valve connects the right atrium with the right ventricle, and another valve connects the left atrium with the left ventricle. The two ventricles are connected to arteries. The artery connected to the right ventricle leads to the lungs and is called the lung artery. The artery from the left ventricle leads to the body and is called the body artery or aorta. The valves prevent the blood from streaming back to the heart (see figure 6.1). The pacemaker of the heart is the so-called sinus node, which determines the rhythm of the heart. This node issues an electric impulse that spreads via the heart walls. This impulse makes the heart contract: first the atrium, and then the ventricle. During this contraction, blood is pumped into the body. At rest,

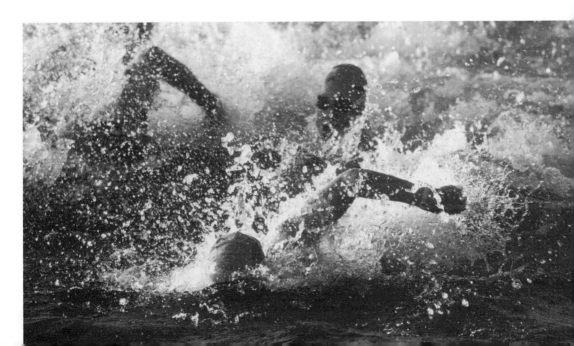

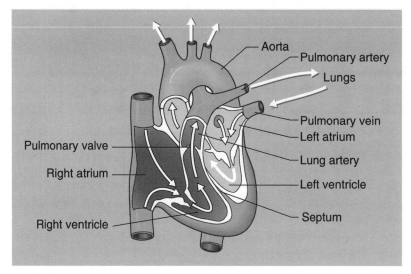

Figure 6.1 The heart.

the heart of untrained persons contracts 60 to 70 times per minute, but during exercise this may rise to 160 to 220 times per minute, depending on age.

The blood that returns to the right atrium is 75% saturated during rest and 20% saturated during heavy exercise. From the atrium on back, the blood is led into the ventricle and then into the lung artery. Within the lungs, carbon dioxide is released and oxygen is loaded into the blood. This oxygen-loaded blood streams into the left atrium and left ventricle from where the blood is pumped into the body via the aorta. To perform all this heavy work, the heart itself also needs blood, which is supplied via a system of arteries around the heart called the coronary arteries.

In the last few decades it has become obvious that intensive endurance sports are not bad for the heart. With regular exercise, the heart adapts to the heavy workload and functions efficiently during heavy exertion.

Favorable Health Effects of Exercise

Sports training has many favorable effects. Obesity diminishes, and the amount of body fat decreases. The total triglyceride and cholesterol levels diminish, and the proportion of high-density lipoprotein (HDL) cholesterol increases. This is favorable, because HDL cholesterol protects the body against cardiovascular diseases. The proportion of low-density lipoprotein cholesterol, which does not have this cardioprotective effect, decreases. Capillarization of the heart muscle improves with exercise, and blood pressure decreases. Sports training combined with a controlled diet favorably affects diabetes. Participation in sport activities usually is accompanied by a healthy lifestyle; people who exercise regularly, rarely smoke, and drink little or no alcohol. People who exercise tend to handle stress more effectively, because sport provides an outlet for them. For all of these reasons, sports participation enhances a person's quality of life.

Cardiovascular Disease

Because inactivity causes a distinct deterioration of heart muscle function, lack of exercise is one of the risk factors for cardiovascular diseases. In healthy young men, a deterioration of the heart function by 10% to 15% was found after a period of bed rest. This deterioration was biggest in those who had the highest maximal oxygen consumption ($\dot{V}O_2$max) and the highest heart volume before the period of bed rest.

Lack of exercise in combination with overweight is a major health problem in the western world. More than half the deaths in the United States are because of cardiovascular diseases. A person who is considerably overweight runs a 2.5 times higher risk of dying because of cardiovascular problems. An important cause of morbid obesity is lack of exercise. Regular physical activities diminish obesity and lower the chance of developing cardiovascular diseases. Following are the three most important risk factors for a heart attack:

- Smoking
- High blood pressure
- High cholesterol level

If all three factors are present, the person's chance of a heart attack is multiplied by 5.

When the heart is taxed repeatedly during regular exercise, the cavities will enlarge and the muscle wall will grow thicker. This enables more blood to be pumped in one stroke. A heart that has undergone such adaptations is called a sports heart, which, contrary to opinions of a short time ago, is a normal physiological adaptation to regular physical exercise.

Women run a lower risk than men of acute cardiac problems during exercise or some hours later. Middle-aged women have fewer ischemic heart failures than men of the same age. This is because in addition to smoking less, women have 25% higher levels of HDL cholesterol than men, a benefit related to the hormone estrogen. Sports participation positively affects HDL cholesterol concentration, as do reduction of body weight and giving up smoking. Every milligram increase of HDL concentration per deciliter of blood decreases the risk of ischemic heart disease by 2% to 3%.

The Heart Minute Volume

The heart minute volume (HMV) is the quantity of blood the heart pumps out in 1 minute. The formula is as follows:

$$HMV = SV \times HR$$

where HMV = milliliters of blood the heart pumps out per minute, SV = stroke volume, and HR = heart rate.

Whenever oxygen supply in working muscle cells is limited, their aerobic endurance capacity diminishes. An endurance athlete with anemia is not capable of transporting sufficient oxygen to the muscle cells. For such an athlete, aerobic energy production will stall sooner, and acidosis will come about more quickly. But the body is capable of adapting itself to the greater oxygen demand. As a result of training, within the muscle cell the number of enzymes necessary to oxidize fatty acids and carbohydrates will increase. These enzyme systems within the muscle cells are "energy factories," which obtain more output capacity through training and therefore are capable of supplying more aerobic energy for a longer period of time. The heart also adapts to training. By just enlarging SV by 25% or even 50%, the capacity of oxygen transport increases enormously.

Stroke Volume

In nonathletes, the heart will beat faster during exercise. In athletes doing the same exercise, the heart will pump more strongly, because the enlarged left ventricle will pump out more blood per stroke. So by just increasing the volume of the left ventricle, HR will remain considerably lower.

Comparison of nonathlete and athlete

Nonathlete: Stroke volume = 90 milliliters

Resting HR (HRrest) = 75 beats per minute (bpm)

Maximum HR (HRmax) = 180 bpm

Resting HMV (HMVrest) = 6,750 milliliters per minute

Maximum HMV (HMVmax) = 16,200 milliliters per minute

Endurance athlete: Stroke volume = 200 milliliters

HRrest = 40 bpm

HRmax = 180 bpm

HMVrest = 8,000 milliliters per minute

HMVmax = 36,000 milliliters per minute

These examples show the enormous changes and adaptations caused by regular exercise. The SV of an endurance athlete at rest is somewhat lower than 200 milliliters. During physical exercise, volume will increase gradually up to a maximum of 200 milliliters.

Starting from a hemoglobin level of 15 grams per 100 milliliters of blood, the maximum oxygen transport of the nonathlete is 3,256 milliliters of oxygen per minute. The endurance athlete reaches 7,236 milliliters of blood per minute. The heart volume decreases in the transition from a lying to an upright position, and performance capacity is diminished. For example, cyclists sit in a bent position because this improves their aerodynamics but also because it is the position in which their heart volumes are bigger. During maximal ergometer tests, HR often decreases at the moment the person bends down to the drops of the handlebars.

Men have a larger SV than women, because the cardiac output per heartbeat has a larger volume in men. The HMV for men is 10% to 20% higher, whereas HRmax is the same for men and women. Training also enlarges the female heart and with that increases stroke volume, but the difference between men and women cannot be compensated for completely by training.

The Sports Heart

Oxygen transport to the working muscles is one of the decisive factors in the ability to perform heavy muscular work. The muscles must receive enough oxygen to oxidize carbohydrates and fatty acids. Within the muscle cells, the enzymes need oxygen in the oxidation processes. Training enlarges the capacity of these enzyme systems. In other words, as a result of training, the muscle cells can handle more oxygen and therefore supply more energy.

The cardiovascular system plays an important role in the transport of oxygen to the working muscles. During long endurance workouts, the heart undergoes certain changes, which include an increase in the heart's size. There has been much discussion about whether heart enlargement caused by endurance exercise is a physiological change. Some scientists have believed that long and exhausting endurance work might rapidly deteriorate the heart muscle. In the 19th century, there was even the misconception that life expectancy was shorter for athletes than for nonathletes.

Even as late as the 1950s, researchers wrote that a sports heart must be a "sick" heart. As knowledge about the sports heart increased, it became clear that the heart's adaptations in response to exercise are practically always of a physiological nature and have nothing to do with heart disease. Through new methods of investigation, especially echocardiography, insight is growing. But there are still many questions, primarily because it is not always easy to distinguish between a sports heart and a heart that is enlarged because of disease. Jumping to rapid and unfounded conclusions has made patients out of many healthy athletes. It is for this reason that the subject—although it is a specialty field—is discussed in this book.

Changes in the Cardiovascular System in Endurance Sports

Endurance sports increase the HMV. A well-trained cyclist reaches an HMV of about 35 liters of blood per minute. Untrained persons reach only 20 liters. In endurance sports, the heart has to handle a large volume of blood input, which means a chronic volume overburdening. Another striking change brought about by training is that the morning pulse decreases. In extremely well-trained athletes, a morning HR less than 30 is no exception. This decrease of the morning pulse comes about under the influence of the involuntary nervous system. The involuntary nervous system consists of a sympathetic and a parasympathetic part, between which there is a certain equilibrium. Endurance training makes the parasympathetic part of the nervous system dominant. This influences the nervus vagus (vagabond nerve), the nerve that sets the HR. On the other hand, the HRmax remains unchanged or decreases slightly in extremely well-trained athletes.

So the HMVrest remains the same or decreases slightly because of more effective oxygen consumption in the muscles. The heart gradually increases in size, and through chronic overburdening the volume of the left ventricle increases. The thickness of the septum (the partition wall between the left and right ventricle) and of the back of the left ventricle increases, resulting in optimum tension of the heart walls. The larger left ventricle, the larger stroke volume, and the lower heart rate are all consequences of endurance training.

Sports that may result in an enlarged heart

Endurance sports	Power sports
Running	Weight lifting
Cycling	Bodybuilding
Swimming	Shot-putting
Cross-country skiing	Discus throwing

The Sports Heart in Endurance Sports

Endurance sports result in a great demand for oxygen in the working muscles. The large HMV results in a chronic volume over stressing of the heart, which causes the heart to adapt itself. The heart's volume increases, and the muscle walls thicken in order to maintain tension, because otherwise the heart would be big and feeble. Volume is most important in the sports heart caused by endurance sports.

The Sports Heart in Power Sports

Power sports cause a strong increase in blood pressure during exercise, which causes a chronic pressure overburdening of the heart. This makes the heart muscle grow thicker, but the cavities do not enlarge much. The most important characteristic of the sports heart in power sports is an increase in muscle mass of the heart.

The Cyclist's Heart

Recent investigations suggest that the cyclist's heart shows the properties of a power sports heart. Although investigations still continue, it seems clear that in the last few years, cycling has evolved into a power sport.

Cyclists also often have a vascular condition called *stenosis arteria iliaca*, which is a thickening of the arteria iliaca externa, a rather common but little-known profession-related illness. The aorta that springs from the heart runs in front of the spine. At the height of the top of the pelvic bone, at the level of the navel, this aorta divides into two arteries: the right and left arteria iliaca communis. Both arteria iliacae communes divide into the arteria iliaca interna, which supplies blood to the smaller pelvis and the musculus psoas, and an arteria iliaca externa, which runs under the ligamentum inguinale, in the groin, to the leg. The anatomy of the arteria iliaca externa and the specific posture of cyclists together with the cycling motion are the most important factors that give rise to this complaint.

During cycling, with its repetitive hip flexion, the arteria iliaca externa is repeatedly kinked. Because of repetitive mechanical stress, a fibrous thickening of the artery wall will result. During strenuous cycling events such as climbing, time trials, or sprinting, the blood supply to the leg literally may be blocked and the rider will find that maximum effort is no longer possible.

In the last few years, hundreds of cyclists with a stenosis of the arteria iliaca externa have undergone surgery. This mainly occurs in high-level riders (professional riders and top amateurs) who have practiced their sport for several years. The problem occurs in the left leg twice as much as in the right, and it occasionally is found bilaterally. The surgical results are generally good.

Characteristics of the Sports Heart

The items discussed next require rather special knowledge. However, to provide a total picture of the sports heart, this information cannot be left out.

Sports heart characteristics

- A slow pulse
- A heart murmur in 40% of cases
- Increased heart volume

In addition, different patterns of electrocardiogram (ECG) may show the following:

- Bradycardia may be present, a pronounced slow heart rate at rest with a minimum of 25 beats per minute.

- A nondangerous irregularity of the heart rhythm is present in 60% of the cases.
- Atrium fluttering may be present, periods of rhythm irregularities that are dangerous. These periods occur at unexpected moments, and therefore a diagnosis is difficult.
- Heart block may be present. Due to the slow heart rate at rest, 10% of cases have a Wenckebach first- or second-degree arteriovenous block. This conductivity disorder is closely related to the intensity of training, and it disappears after stopping exercise.

ECG Irregularities

Left ventricle enlargement is noticeable on the ECG of a sports heart and is more often seen in endurance athletes than in power athletes. The ECG may show an incomplete right bundle-branch block, which is caused by the increased muscle mass at the tip of the heart. Ten percent of endurance athletes have an abnormal ST segment (which is a segment of the ECG reading). There is no explanation for this phenomenon, but it is widely believed that this disturbance does not indicate a disordered heart muscle. During light physical exercise this abnormal ST segment completely disappears, which is a sign that the abnormal ST segment does not indicate a sick heart. In patients with a sick heart, abnormalities become more distinct during exercise.

Abnormalities on the ECG at rest often cannot be distinguished from an acute heart attack. If the cardiologist who views the ECG does not know that the person is an athlete, he or she will immediately assume that the person has a heart disorder or is having a heart attack. Jumping to rapid and unfounded conclusions has turned many healthy athletes into patients.

Well-trained endurance athletes may reach a muscle wall of the left ventricle of maximally 13 millimeters. A wall thickness more than 13 millimeters indicates a morbid heart enlargement. In endurance athletes, there is a normal relationship between muscle mass and heart volume; thus, the mass/volume ratio is normal. In power athletes, only the muscle mass of the ventricle has increased by 30% to 70%, which increases the mass/volume ratio.

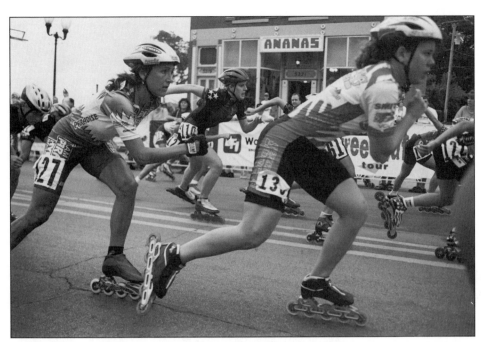

Skating has many of the same cardiovascular effects as cycling.

If endurance training is maintained, the heart does not continue to enlarge. It seems that the heart has a built-in protective mechanism against overburdening. Yet much research is still needed to determine the effects of long-term endurance exercise. I believe that extreme endurance sports, such as the Tour de France, damage health in general and the heart in particular.

The athlete's heart remains enlarged after his or her career ends. The heart may decrease somewhat, but it will never be a normal heart again. There are no indications that at a later age people with a sports heart experience more heart problems than those who have never done any physical exercise.

The enlarged sports heart is a normal physiological adaptation, but many questions about the sports heart remain unanswered. For that matter, it is not known why not all endurance athletes develop a sports heart. A trained athlete who does not have a sports heart may perform excellently. Extremely few cyclists have a sports heart. Possibly, developing a sports heart depends on predisposition and hereditary factors.

chapter 7

Blood Levels

If oxygen transport diminishes, for whatever reason, heart rate (HR) increases in an attempt to maintain the level of oxygen transport. This increased HR decreases performance capacity, so a well-functioning oxygen transport system is essential for top performance.

Characteristics of Blood

An adult has about 5 liters of blood. Blood consists of two components: blood plasma and blood cells. The blood plasma is a clear, yellowish liquid in which the blood cells are dissolved. Red blood cells make up 40% to 45% of the total quantity of blood. This percentage is called the hematocrit (Hct) level of the blood. Normal Hct levels are 40% to 54% for males and 37% to 50% for females.

Most blood cells are red blood cells, also called erythrocytes. The lifespan of erythrocytes is about 90 days. Every cubic milliliter of blood contains 4 to 6 million red blood cells. The red color of the blood is caused by a ferrous protein called hemoglobin (Hb).

Hb may bind oxygen and transport it from the lungs to the muscle cells. One gram of Hb may bind 1.34 milliliters of oxygen. Men have an average of 15 grams of Hb per 100 milliliters (i.e., 1 deciliter) of blood; women have 12 grams per 100 milliliters. So in men, 100 milliliters of blood may transport

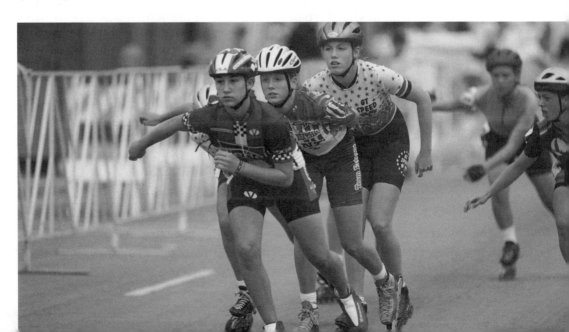

$1.34 \times 15 = 20$ milliliters of oxygen; in women, $1.34 \times 12 = 16$ milliliters of oxygen.

Because Hb content in men is about 10% higher than in women, women's oxygen transport capacity is lower. Moreover, many female athletes balance on the brink of anemia because of blood loss during menstruation, iron loss from exercise itself, and limited nutrition. In female athletes, anemia attributable to iron deficiency is rather common.

Exercising women have an increased need for iron. Iron, which is lost in sweat, urine, and monthly menstruation, is essential for building up Hb. An iron deficiency diminishes immunity against infections. Recovery after a race or strenuous workout will be slower in athletes who have poor iron status. A pronounced iron deficiency diminishes performance capacity and leads to fatigue. The athlete should take in sufficient iron with everyday food, by eating many vegetables, red meat, and whole-wheat products. Drinking coffee, tea, and milk with meals should be avoided because these products inhibit iron absorption. Instead, it is better to drink fruit juices with meals. Sometimes, in cases of pronounced iron deficiency, the athlete may need iron supplementation. However, people should take iron supplements only when blood tests indicate an iron deficiency, because too much iron within the body can be harmful.

Normal Hb levels for males are 8.7 to 10.9 millimoles per liter, or 13.9 to 17.4 grams per 100 milliliters (grams per deciliter); for females, Hb levels are 7.5 to 9.7 millimoles per liter or 12.0 to 15.5 grams per 100 milliliters (grams per deciliter). The conversion formula is millimoles $\times 1.6$ = grams per 100 milliliters.

The red blood cells bind and transport oxygen. If Hb decreases from 10 to 9 millimoles per liter, the blood will be capable of transporting 10% less oxygen. Maximal oxygen uptake ($\dot{V}O_2$max) then decreases by about 10%, because it depends largely on oxygen transport capacity. When oxygen transport is diminished, performance capacity decreases as well. In this situation, the body has to switch to anaerobic energy supply, and lactate is formed at an earlier stage. When Hb decreases, the HR increases, because the heart must circulate more blood to maintain the same level of oxygen transport.

Decrease in Oxygen Transport

Possible causes for decreased oxygen transport capacity of the blood that might be important to athletes are blood loss, lack of oxygen in the air, blockade of Hb, and anemia.

Blood Loss

In the case of blood loss, oxygen transport capacity diminishes. Many athletes regularly donate blood at blood banks, usually 0.5 liters of blood each time. After such a donation it takes 3 to 4 weeks before the Hb level returns to the previous value. During this period the athlete has diminished capacity to perform at maximum level. So it is inadvisable to donate blood 3 to 4 weeks before an important race.

Lack of Oxygen

At a high altitude, the quantity of oxygen in the air decreases. At about 1,800 meters elevation, people from sea level notice a lack of oxygen. This decreases performance capacity during the first few days of a stay at a high altitude, while the body takes time to acclimatize. The lack of oxygen stimulates the bone marrow to generate more red blood cells, which is why the Hb levels of people living in higher areas are distinctly higher than those of lowlanders. After a stay of 2 to 3 weeks at a higher altitude, that athlete may have the subjective feeling that he can resume training activities with low level intensity again. His HRrest has gone back to normal. Acclimatization may then be considered complete. Training at a high altitude requires adaptation, which may take 8 to 14 days. By checking the morning pulse, the athlete can determine the degree of adaptation.

Altitude deserves serious consideration in planning a training program. The pace that the athlete used at sea level will cause a higher HR at altitude. Recovery after workouts during the adaptation period requires more time. Both the volume and the intensity of training should be decreased at altitude until acclimatization is complete. If extra time is not devoted to recovery, fatigue will accumulate and extra rest will be necessary before normal training can be resumed. In training camps at higher altitudes, there is always the danger that athletes become overfatigued and overtrained. In the beginning Hb level may increase by 1% per week, but this increase slowly diminishes after a 12-week stay at a high altitude, Hb may have increased by as much as 10%.

When training in high altitudes, the athlete should be sure that his or her iron supplies are sufficient and should consume extra iron in case of deficits. The ideal altitude for altitude training is 2,000 to 2,500 meters. Endurance athletes require a minimum of 3 weeks to become acclimatized, although 4 to 6 weeks is ideal. At the beginning of altitude training, the workouts should be limited and then can be extended gradually. The athlete should not force workouts, certainly not in the first few days. The athlete should pay extra attention to rest and recovery, to warming up and cooling down, to nutrition, and to the risk of sunburn. After returning to sea level, an acclimatization period of 5 days is advisable before the athlete resumes racing. The best performances may be expected 7 to 10 days after returning to sea level. But the positive effect lasts much longer, because the lifespan of red blood cells is 90 days.

Altitude training may be simulated by the use of low-pressure chambers (hypobaric chambers). Within these chambers the air pressure is lowered, thus lowering partial oxygen pressure.

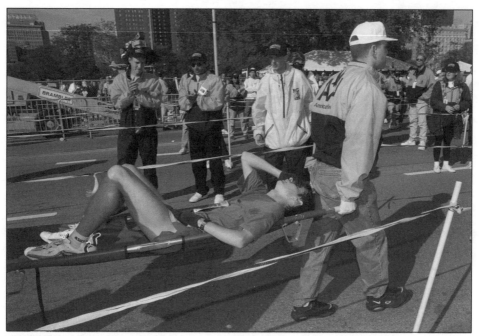

Too little oxygen overstrains the muscles and quickly causes collapse.

Blockade of Hb

One of the disadvantages of smoking is that carbon monoxide (CO) is bound to the Hb in the blood, which has a major impact on physical capacity. CO is bound to Hb about 200 times as fast as oxygen, so only a small quantity of CO is required to distinctly deteriorate the oxygen-loading capacity of the blood. Smoking just one cigarette results in about 5% of the Hb being bound to carbon monoxide. This strong binding of CO to Hb means that it takes many hours for the CO to dissipate. Heavy smokers often have more than 15% of their Hb bound to CO. The decline of oxygen content in the blood will decrease maximum oxygen consumption and therefore physical capacity.

Smoking is not the only source of CO. Exhaust fumes from motor vehicles contain large quantities of CO. Therefore, it is inadvisable to train in heavy traffic, for example, along a highway. In races, runners and cyclists can be impeded by following cars and motorcycles. Just think of cyclists in the Tour de France climbing a mountain slope. They are surrounded by a swarm of motorcycles, at the very moment that they are performing maximally. The CO intake in such a situation must be considerable. For example, on a motorway in Los Angeles, an average CO of 5 parts per million is measured. One hour on or near that highway, even at rest, results in CO concentration in the blood as high as 3%. After 8 hours, this percentage is 8%.

During physical exercise breathing is faster, which increases CO concentration in the blood even more quickly. At a CO concentration of 6% and greater, some serious problems may occur such as impaired vision, slowed reaction, and decreased performance capacity. A 6% CO concentration in the blood is reached after 1 hour of exposure, at rest, to air that contains 100 parts of CO per million. This concentration is often measured in Los Angeles in tunnels or near traffic lights. The accepted value of CO in Los Angeles is 35 parts per million. If this limit is surpassed, the local authorities give advice to limit CO output.

Anemia

Endurance athletes often suffer from anemia, which is caused by lack of iron. Characteristics of anemia include lower levels of Hb, serum iron, and ferritin. Women are especially susceptible to anemia because of monthly menstruation. The classic symptoms of anemia in nonathletes are fatigue, dizziness, impaired vision, palpitations, and paleness. Nonathletes have these complaints when Hb is lower than 6.5 millimoles per liter.

Athletes feel their complaints sooner and their complaints are different from those of sedentary people. Performance level decreases, and the athlete has excessive fatigue after a workout or race. The athlete may have sore legs when walking or cycling, or even when climbing stairs. Very often the athlete feels soreness during accelerations. The day after a race the athlete is often tired, with a higher morning pulse. If an athlete's Hb decreases from 9.0 to 8.0 millimoles per liter, his or her oxygen transport capacity decreases by more than 10%. Acidosis will sooner occur after a decrease in Hb. In cases of anemia, Hb is the last parameter to decrease. Iron not only is an essential factor for Hb but is also closely connected to all kinds of metabolic processes. Iron deficiency is a matter not only of diminished oxygen transport but also of insufficient energy supply.

There are multiple causes of iron deficiency in endurance athletes. The diet may contain insufficient iron, and the nutritional pattern may play a role. Tea and coffee interfere with iron absorption. Vitamin C, taken together with iron or ferrous nutrients, furthers iron absorption, so a vitamin C deficiency can contribute to iron deficiency.

Perspiration during exercise may cause extra iron loss. In addition, red blood cells may be damaged because of a mechanical or chemical trauma, a condition called hemolysis. Mechanical trauma is caused when running; every footstrike is a blow to the sole of the foot, which damages red blood cells and shortens their lifespan. Chemical trauma, which is caused by lack of oxygen or heightened lactate values of free oxygen radicals, also shortens the lifespan of red blood cells.

Extreme endurance efforts may cause minor hemorrhages in the bowels and bladder, resulting in blood loss via feces and urine. Toxic conditions such as infections and consequently the circulating toxic substances may cause a chronic hemolytic aspect. Notorious are chronic tonsillitis, chronic sinusitis, and inflamed teeth roots, but other infections may also be the cause.

To maintain performance, iron deficits should be avoided. Several steps will help to avoid such deficits. Nutrition should be varied, and the athlete should avoid drinking tea or coffee with meals. Athletes should consume products rich in iron, such as parsley, broad beans, lamb's lettuce, kidney beans, marrowfat peas and lentils, brown bread, whole-wheat bread, apple sauce, molasses, liver, pork, and beef. Athletes also should consume vitamin C via fruit, vegetables, potatoes, and fruit juices.

Endurance athletes who train many hours should have their Hb, serum iron, and ferritin levels checked regularly. If an iron deficit should occur, it may be necessary to take iron supplements.

Iron Therapy

In sports the custom is to inject iron into a vein (intravenously) or into a muscle (intramuscularly). The idea behind this is that injections might refill the body deficits sooner compared with oral intake. But this is a misconception, because administering iron by injecting it does not lead to a more rapid production of red blood cells. If iron is administered by injection, this certainly should not be combined with oral intake.

Iron injections are potentially dangerous and may have unfavorable complications. Hypersensitivity reactions occur, though rarely, with both intravenous and intramuscular injections. They may be serious, and even a few deaths are reported. Such a reaction occurs in the first few minutes after the injection and is characterized by breathing difficulty and shock. Immediate hypersensitivity is also manifested by a rash, itching, nausea, and shivers. If these complications appear, the administration should be stopped immediately. Some delayed reactions also are reported that can be dangerous. These reactions are more common after large doses are administered intravenously, but they also can occur after intramuscular injections. Characteristic of these reactions are sore joints and muscles and sometimes fever, which may be seen from some hours to 4 days after the injection. These flu-like symptoms last 2 to 4 days and then disappear spontaneously or after administration of a simple analgesic. Furthermore, there may be pain and inflammation at the spot of the injection. With the wrong injection technique a brownish spot may occur, which remains for life.

A paramedical attendant once administered a monthly iron injection to an athlete. The result was that the athlete had flu-like symptoms for 2 to 4 days every month. Not surprisingly, his performance was rather poor. The touches of flu disappeared after the injections were stopped, and he even won a few important races. So my advice is to avoid iron injections even when a deficit is obvious.

Hemochromatosis

A large store of iron within the body may create a rather dangerous situation for the athlete, in the form of hemochromatosis. Primary hemochromatosis, the hereditary form of this disease, is rather common in men. Secondary hemochromatosis can be caused by excessive iron intake, via either supplements or injections, so athletes may have this illness. Many doctors believe that hemochromatosis is a rare disease, so it often is misdiagnosed or is diagnosed too late, when the illness is in the later stages and there is extensive organ damage.

Routine blood checks in professional athletes, especially cyclists, often show high serum ferritin values; more than 500 micrograms per liter is not exceptional. Normal ferritin values are between 18 and 370 micrograms per liter for men.

Under normal conditions the body contains 3 to 4 grams of iron. The daily loss of iron, which is about 1 milligram per day, is replenished by iron absorption out of nutrition in the intestines. When the iron supply in nutrition increases greatly, it will not automatically lead to more absorption; only when there is an iron deficit will the intestines absorb more, because of a regulative system in the intestines that prevents overabsorption.

There are two types of hemochromatosis: the primary or hereditary type and the secondary or developed type. Primary hemochromatosis is caused by a defective gene on chromosome 6, causing an abnormal absorption and storage of iron from the intestines. When ferritin is fully saturated with iron, the storage of iron bound to ferritin is no longer possible. Then the surplus of iron must be stored in the heart, liver, pancreas, pituitary and adrenal glands, testes, kidneys, and joints.

Hereditary hemochromatosis is rather common. One out of every 10 people carries the defective gene on one chromosome (heterozygous). Three out of every 1,000 people carry the defective gene on both chromosomes (homozygous). In these people, hereditary hemochromatosis may be manifest (see figure 7.1).

Hereditary hemochromatosis can be recessive autosomal. Recessive means that the defective gene is not manifest, and autosomal means that the defective gene is not on the sex chromosomes. Hemochromatosis occurs especially in men, because women lose much iron during menstruation. The diagnosis often is made late in life, often after the 50th year, because the symptoms of the illness are rather nonspecific. On the other hand, patients who do not have any complaints or symptoms may have disturbed iron values in their blood already.

Secondary hemochromatosis can be caused by multiple factors. First is a defect in the formation of Hb or the red blood cell, as occurs in thallasemia,

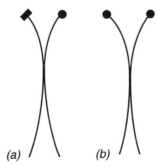

(a)   *(b)*

Figure 7.1 *(a)* **Heterozygous chromosome, note the defective gene,** *(b)* **homozygous chromosome.**

sickle-cell anemia, aplastic anemia, and sideroblastic anemia, conditions that require regular blood transfusions. In case of massive bleeding much iron is lost, and then blood transfusions cannot cause hemochromatosis.

Clinical Symptoms

Athletes suffering from hemochromatosis may exhibit the following symptoms in addition to performance declines:

Liver: liver enlargement, pain in the liver region, liver insufficiency, liver cirrhosis, liver cancer, hemorrhages in the esophagus because of varicose veins

Heart: heart condition, enlargement, tachycardia, fatigue, weight loss

Pancreas: diabetes

Skin: gray because of the iron and brownish because of melanin

Testes: loss of libido and impotence

Joints: painful joints

Diagnosis is made with routine laboratory tests: erythrocyte sedimentation rate, C-reactive protein, Hb, mean cell volume, serum ferritin, transferrin-iron saturation, y gt, and alanine aminotranferase. A progressive increase in transferrin-iron saturation is an excellent indicator for hemochromatosis (serum iron ÷ iron binding capacity × 100) (%). If a progressive increase is established, genetic research is indicated to determine whether it is a case of primary or secondary hemochromatosis.

The ferritin level is a standard for the iron stores in the body. In case of a progressive increase of ferritin level, the possibility of hemochromatosis should always be considered. A strong increase in ferritin level is also symptomatic of other conditions.

With various infections and all acute infections, erythrocyte sedimentation and C-reactive protein are higher. These include the following:

- Pneumonia
- Osteomyelitis
- Chronic urethra infections
- Rheumatic arthritis
- Liver disease
- Chronic viral hepatitis
- Liver damage due to chronic alcohol abuse

Erythrocyte sedimentation and C-reactive protein are also higher in the presence of certain cancers:

- Acute leukemia
- Hodgkin's disease
- Breast cancer

The ferritin determination is less specific than the transferrin-iron saturation determination, but ferritin determination is an ideal and simple way of screening for hemochromatosis, because normal ferritin values exclude hemochromatosis. In cases of higher ferritin values, the blood investigation should be extended until the correct diagnosis is reached.

Genetic investigation is used to determine the type of hemochromatosis that an athlete has. The defective gene on chromosome 6 is not the only explanation for hemochromatosis. In Italy, 70% of the hemochromatosis patients had the defective gene, as expected, but the gene could not detected in the other 30% (Carella 1997). Thus, it is impossible to find all hemochromatosis patients through genetic screening only. The heterozygous people, who make up 10% of the population, mostly have somewhat higher ferritin levels, the average being 370 micrograms per liter. It is impossible to predict through genetic screening whether they will develop hemochromatosis. It is known that heterozygous people run a higher risk of developing hemochromatosis in the case of excessive exogenous iron supply.

In the case of a high ferritin level, the investigation should be repeated after some time to exclude infections. Ferritin testing should be considered to screen systematically for ferritin and transferrin-iron saturation in everybody over 30. In case the second blood sample also shows increased ferritin, the blood investigation should be extended to determine serum iron content and transferrin content. When the transferrin-iron saturation surpasses 60% in men or 50% in women, a genetic investigation should be conducted to confirm the diagnosis. If this genetic test is positive, a liver biopsy should be performed to determine the degree of liver damage.

If a genetic test proves negative there are two possibilities: Hemochromatosis is caused by an unknown genetic defect, or it is caused by excessive exogenous iron supply.

Treatment

Iron supplementation should be stopped immediately. The athlete should undergo weekly bloodletting of 500 milliliters per week, until normal ferritin and Hb values are reached. Five hundred milliliters of blood corresponds to 250 milligrams of iron, so some 15 to 25 grams of iron can be eliminated per year.

A second possibility is an intramuscular injection of the iron chelator desferal, a substance that binds iron. The body excretes the iron and chelator via the kidneys and bilious ducts. This method is capable of expelling 5 to 15 grams of iron per year. If hemochromatosis is found in any patient, all his or her relatives should be screened as well. If the illness is diagnosed and treated before organ damage occurs, life expectancy is normal.

Reference values are listed here. For serum iron, 12 to 35 micromoles per liter is normal for men and 13 to 35 micromoles per liter for women. Serum values greater than 72 for men and greater than 68 for women indicate an excess supply of iron that requires treatment.

For ferritin, 18 to 370 nanograms per milliliter is normal for men and 10 to 120 nanograms per milliliter for women. The reference values of ferritin more or less depend on the laboratory method used. Further analysis of this iron storage is indicated when serum ferritin values surpass 300 (men) and 150 (women) and when hepatitis and iron supplementation are excluded.

For transferrin, 2.0 to 4.0 grams per liter is normal for adults. Transferrin values less than 1.0 gram per liter require further analysis, because these values are low in hemochromatosis patients. Lack of iron shows transferrin values greater than 5.0. For adults, total iron binding capacity is 50 to 78 micromoles per liter.

Optimizing Oxygen Transport

Maximum achievement requires an optimum supply of oxygen sent to the muscles. As oxygen transport improves, Hb content increases and so do $\dot{V}O_2$max and performance capacity. If the red blood cells are not capable of delivering sufficient oxygen, performance will suffer. Ways that athletes attempt to improve oxygen transport, with varying degrees of success, include training at higher altitudes, transfusion of red blood cells (called blood doping), use of devices such as nose strips or hypoxic tents, or a course of erythropoietin (EPO). Athletes who already have a high Hb level will get little benefit from these steps. But usually intensively training endurance athletes have a low Hb level and therefore an insufficient oxygen transport.

Blood Doping

During the 1976 Olympic Games, the Finnish long-distance runner Lasse Viren was accused by the press of blood doping, after he had won both the 5,000-meter and 10,000-meter races and was fifth in the marathon. This achievement was tremendous indeed, and it is small wonder that people wanted to find the "cause." Blood doping—which involves taking blood from someone and reinfusing the same blood after some time—is done to temporarily enlarge blood volume and, most important, to increase the number of red blood cells. The increased Hb level enables the blood to transport more oxygen and thus increases the athlete's aerobic capacity. Scientific research has proven that blood doping does work if the oxygen transport capacity is deficient. In athletes whose oxygen supply to the muscles is optimal, blood doping has no effect. Blood doping mostly uses the athlete's own blood. If someone else's blood were used, certain complications might occur such as transfusion reactions or contamination with viral infections. And with any transfusion there is always the danger of embolism and thrombosis.

Hypoxic Tents

The Belgian cyclist Johan Museeuw sleeps in a hypoxic tent, together with his family. Many other professional riders use hypoxic tents in an attempt to improve their performance. The theory behind the use of such tents is the same as the theory behind altitude training: that a lack of oxygen improves condition.

Mixing more nitrogen in normal air diminishes oxygen pressure. When this mixture is blown into a tent this creates an oxygen-poor atmosphere. For an optimal system, a nitrogen cylinder is necessary, which is rather heavy. This is not very convenient for traveling athletes, who often travel by plane and stay in hotels during the racing season.

The hypoxic tent solves the transport problem and makes oxygen-poor surroundings rather cheap. An electric pump draws air over a membrane, creating an oxygen-poor fraction that is blown into the tent. The athlete who sleeps in these surroundings inhales air with an oxygen content of 15%, which is comparable to an altitude of 3,000 meters but with the normal air pressure. The tent and generator together weigh about 30 kilograms and can be transported in a van. The tent is quickly set up in a hotel room. The cost of the equipment is less than $5,000.

Erythropoietin (EPO)

EPO stimulates the body's production of red blood cells and provides an alternative for altitude training and blood doping, although it is banned by most sports organizations. Under normal physiological conditions, the production of EPO, which takes place in the liver and kidneys, is initiated by the oxygen pressure in the blood. A low oxygen pressure leads to the production of EPO; this EPO stimulates the bone marrow to produce red blood cells, and the oxygen transport capacity of the blood increases.

Normally occurring EPO and recombinant EPO can be distinguished chemically, so the use of exogenous EPO can be detected, although this has not yet led to a watertight doping test for EPO. In testing for the use of exogenous EPO, Hct values give too little information to prove blood manipulation. Erythrocyte volume may be constant while a change in the amount of blood plasma (e.g., through dehydration or infusion) might render a higher, lower, or equal Hct. On the other hand, you could conceal an increase of red blood cells by ensuring that your plasma volume is also increased. The maximum Hct values of 50 for men and 47 for women, as adopted by the International Cycling Union (UCI) for their "health controls," are highly questionable. Not only can this Hct value be manipulated, but there is also sufficient proof that some people, both athletes and nonathletes, exceed 50% naturally. This might be the case especially in athletes who live and train at high altitudes. A recent study by Vergouven, Collee, and Marx showed that as many as 20% of people living at high altitude had an Hct of more than 50%.

The only reliable method to detect a change in the number of erythrocytes is to inject a known amount of labeled red blood cells and then establish the degree of dilution in the total amount of red blood cells within the body.

Little is known about the side effects of exogenous EPO use in elite athletes. The symptoms that were prominently discussed in the press, such as a high blood pressure and an enhanced risk of thrombosis, were seen in the first years that EPO was used in the "natural" target group: hemodialysis patients. It was soon found that gradually administering EPO diminished or even eliminated many side effects. So when EPO is used wisely, that is, when the doses are not too high, the chance of undesired side effects is very low.

Exogenous EPO is produced via the recombinant technique. In principle it is possible to produce unlimited quantities. It can be obtained under the names Eprex (manufactured by Cilag) and Reconorm (manufactured by Boehringer-Mannheim).

Physiology

EPO is the most important hormone for the production of red blood cells. EPO is produced in the liver and kidneys. Red blood cells are produced in the bone marrow (see figure 7.2).

From the pluripotent hematopoietic mother, cell pro-erythroblasts are formed. From these are formed the normoblasts, which still possess a nucleus. When this nucleus is gone, they are called reticulocytes, which develop into erythrocytes within the bone marrow. EPO takes care of an eventual increase of reticulocytes and erythrocytes. The production of EPO itself is influenced by the oxygen pressure of the arterial blood; the production of EPO is heightened at a low oxygen pressure. This phenomenon occurs when the person is at a high altitude or when oxygen intake is otherwise diminished, for example, due to chronic lung diseases.

In patients with kidney disease, the natural production of EPO may be diminished considerably. Therefore these patients develop an anemia with low values for Hb, Hct, and red blood cells. Normally, in healthy persons, the production of EPO is stimulated by low Hct values. In patients with kidney disease this is impossible because the damaged kidneys are not capable of producing sufficient EPO. Therefore, exogenous EPO is administered by injection, which might be considered a substitution therapy.

Administering EPO

Most experience in administering exogenous EPO comes from hemodialysis patients. EPO therapy often results in a spectacular improvement of the hemodialysis patient's condition. EPO also may be effective in treating chronic inflammations, cancers, anemia, and rheumatic arthritis and for treating patients who have had chemotherapy with cisplatin. In hemodialysis patients the optimal dose is an intravenous injection three times per week at 30 to 50 international units per kilogram of body weight. For a person

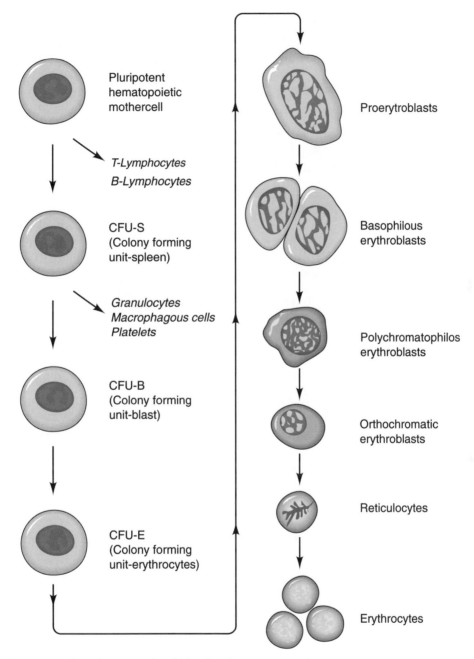

Figure 7.2   Development of red blood cells.

weighing 70 kilograms, this means 2,000 to 3,500 international units at a time. After a week of treatment, Hb, and red blood cells already show increases. Also the number of reticulocytes in the blood increases. The normal values for Hct are 40% to 54% for men and 37% to 50% for women. In hemodialysis patients, the target Hct value is 35%.

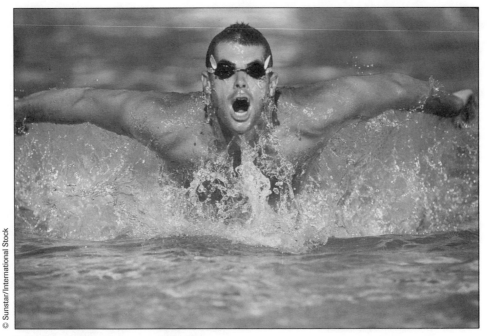

© Sunstar/International Stock

Regular exercise enlarges cardiac output.

When the therapy is started with higher doses, Hct, Hb, and red blood cells increase more rapidly. In the consecutive treatments, doses often are reduced to lower maintenance doses. A good alternative for the intravenous injection is subcutaneous administration. The same therapeutic effect can be reached with a dose reduction of 30% when EPO is administered subcutaneously. So this way of injecting may save 30% of the doses and still have the same effect. During EPO therapy, extra iron, folic acid, and vitamin B_{12} are often given, because these substances play an important role in the formation of red blood cells. During the EPO therapy, the blood should be screened regularly because these blood parameters should not increase too much in a short period of time.

Many side effects are associated with the administration of EPO:

- An increase in blood pressure occurs in 25% of kidney patients. This increase does not occur in patients without kidney problems.

- Thrombosis may occur on the spot of vascular injection, another reason for subcutaneous injections.

Other side effects *after* the injection may include the following:

- Pseudo-flu syndrome
- Pain in the bones
- Cold shivers
- Skin reactions

- Palpebral edema
- Increased appetite

The most important side effects occur when Hct increases too rapidly. The side effects will diminish when the doses are lowered. In kidney patients, cerebrovascular problems and insults are seen as a result of EPO administration. Cardiovascular side effects also are possible, which can be limited by simultaneously administering acetosal.

EPO Use in Sports

EPO, which enhances the body's oxygen supply, is the pharmaceutical alternative for altitude training and for blood doping. In the case of EPO use, the athlete's blood should be screened weekly and the following parameters tested: Hb, Hct, red blood cells, ferritin, and serum iron. Any athlete who chooses to use EPO should seek the help of an experienced doctor.

It is not clear exactly what Hct is optimal for physical exercise, but 50% to 55% is probably close to the ideal figure. An extremely high Hct will not enhance performance, because the more viscose blood will inhibit oxygen transport.

EPO is one of the few pharmaceutical aids that enhance the achievements of cyclists and other endurance athletes. A good cyclist turns into a potential champion by using EPO. Oxygen uptake improves by 8%, and the duration of a considerable effort improves by 16%.

The use of EPO is forbidden by the International Olympic Committee and the UCI. But EPO cannot be detected well by the doping laboratories, because EPO is washed out within 24 hours after the injection. However, the effects of the EPO course can be seen and traced till minimally 4 weeks after an EPO course. A standard EPO course takes 3 to 5 weeks, in which the athlete gets an EPO injection two to three times a week. The performance-enhancing effects start after 1 week and will last 2 to 4 weeks after the athlete finishes the course. After 2 to 4 weeks, the $\dot{V}O_2$max and Hct will return to normal.

Injected EPO can be distinguished from the body's own EPO. As early as 1995, clinical chemists of the University of Uppsala, Sweden, published a urine test to distinguish between injected EPO and natural EPO. In addition, electrophoresis may show these differences.

Hematology specialists think that monthly blood sampling might be the key to prove EPO use. These inexpensive monthly tests measure simple blood values. However, these samples are stored for further and more expensive analysis when the results of the initial, simple tests are suspicious. It is then possible to distinguish between EPO use and the effects of altitude training.

It is hard to understand why altitude training and hypoxic tents are permitted and EPO is not. But the fact is that EPO use is forbidden, and once organizations establish this rule they have a duty to ensure that every athlete has an equal and reasonable chance of being caught. This means a considerable investment in watertight controls based on the present knowledge. When the UCI introduced health controls in 1997, these controls turned out to be a license to increase Hct up to just below 50% through EPO. Reference values for Hct levels of elite athletes are 43% to 51% for men and 38% to 46% for women (see figure 7.3).

EPO Myths

For years there has been an ongoing discussion about the 18 cyclists in The Netherlands and Belgium who died allegedly because of EPO use. Bert Oosterbosch, Connie Meyer, and Johannes Draayer are just a few names. But this scandalous media story is simply untrue. These tragic deaths all occurred during the late 1980s and early 1990s, a time when EPO was not used yet. EPO was introduced in the world of cycling in 1991-1992, and from then its use gradually increased, parallel to the tremendous supremacy of the Italian riders. But if EPO was really as dangerous as alleged, many riders would have died from 1991 to 1997, because the use of EPO was unlimited and uncontrolled before January 1997. After January 1997, when the UCI introduced the 50% Hct measure, the use of EPO became widespread. The 50% Hct measure turned out to be a license to enhance Hct levels up to just under 50%, and the only means that can effectively achieve that end is EPO. So this UCI step stimulated rather than restricted the use of EPO. The extreme peaks in Hct values that were seen before January 1997 have since disappeared. The 18 deaths would have nothing to do with this EPO story if they were not constantly used as an argument to intensify the campaign against doping in general and EPO in particular.

Another myth about EPO is that the higher an athlete's Hct level, the higher his or her $\dot{V}O_2$max will be and consequently the better performance will be. This is also not true. There is an optimum for Hct values and consequent oxygen transport and performance capacity. The Danish Tour de France winner Bjarne Riis was called "Monsieur 60%," but it is most unlikely that he would have performed so well with an Hct level of 60 or even higher. When the viscosity of the blood increases too much, its oxygen transport capacity decreases and the cyclist cannot even stay in the pack.

Thirteen long-distance runners trained and lived at an altitude of 2,500 meters. This was the high-high group. Thirteen other distance runners lived at an altitude of 2,500 meters but they trained at 1,250 meters. This was the high-low group. Thirteen other runners remained low as a control group. This was the low-low group. After this altitude period they ran a 5-kilometer race.

The high-low group ran an average of 13 seconds faster than the average of all the 39 runners before the experiment. The high-high group was 17 seconds slower, and the low-low group performed nearly 40 seconds slower. It was striking that the blood values in the high-high group and the high-low group reached the same high levels: Their Hct rose by 10%.

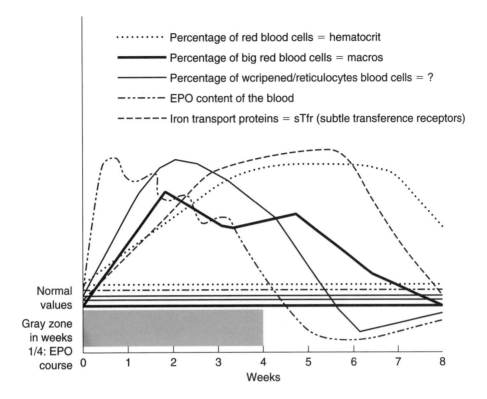

Figure 7.3 Changes caused by the EPO course.

Testing for EPO

The Medical Commission of the International Olympics Committee announced before the start of the Olympic Games in Sydney that they would start testing for the banned substance EPO on September 1, 2000. The tests would especially be targeted toward endurance athletes, such as cyclists, rowers, triathletes, and marathon runners.

The complete EPO test, which works both during the EPO course and during 4 weeks after the last injection, consists of a blood and a urine test. The blood test is an indirect method that makes the first selection. A positive blood test does not directly show injected EPO but rather indicates the likely use of exogenous EPO, because of the effects that EPO causes. By just inspecting various blood values, the use of EPO can be detected.

During the period of EPO use, a combination of blood values betrays that use. These five parameters change during the course:

- The percentage of red blood cells (Hct)
- EPO content of the blood
- Percentage of unripened blood cells (% macros)
- Iron transport protein (soluble transferrin receptors)
- Percentage of large red blood cells (Hct of reticulocytes)

Reticulocytes are the forerunners of the red blood cells. Iron transport proteins ensure that sufficient iron circulates in the blood to make new red blood cells. These five parameters are all heightened during an EPO course.

In the 4 weeks after the EPO course, another combination of blood parameters will betray EPO use. After the course three parameters will change:

- Percentage of red blood cells (Hct)
- Percentage of large red blood cells (Hct of reticulocytes)
- EPO concentration

After the course Hct is heightened, but reticulocytes Hct and EPO level are clearly lower. The blood test detects 94% to 100% of EPO users during the course. In the 4 weeks after the course, the chance of being caught changes. Between the 12th and the 21st day after the last injection, the chance of being caught is 67% to 72%. On the 28th day after the last injection, the chance of being caught is 33% (figure 7.4).

When the blood test is positive, the doping controllers must prove the presence of exogenous EPO in the urine of the athlete; however, the presence of EPO in urine disappears after a few days, and the effects on endurance capacity still remain. If the urine test is also positive, the athlete is found positive and will be suspended. The urine test was developed in France and it is considered a reliable method. The blood tests were developed in Australia and they are not completely watertight in the legal sense. That is the reason why the two tests are both used. As the situation stands, the athlete may stop the course 3 to 5 days before the doping test; the athlete's

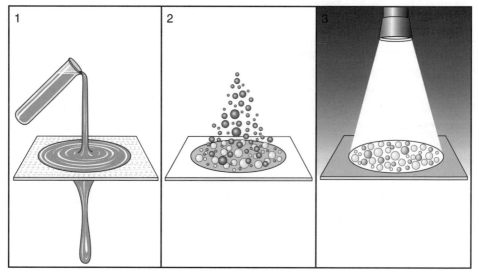

Figure 7.4 EPO urine test.

blood test will be positive but the decisive urine test will be negative again, and the athlete will not be suspended.

In the first step of the urine test, 20 milliliters of urine is filtered. The smaller particles pass the filter. The bigger particles such as EPO and larger proteins are separated by the filter. In the second step, antibodies are added, which attach themselves to EPO and make EPO visible. In the third step, the concentration thus obtained is lit up. Because natural EPO is more acid than artificial EPO, there will be a difference in color and the artificial EPO will be detected (figure 7.4).

During the Olympic Games of Sydney, no athlete was caught using EPO. This is logical, because the urine test must supply decisive proof of the use of EPO. But positive blood tests must have been found. It seems that the EPO era is drawing to an end. It remains questionable whether that is something to be optimistic about, because new drugs to stimulate red blood cell production are being developed.

The protein that stimulates the production of natural EPO in hypoxic surroundings has been found. This "hypoxia-associated factor" stimulates the gene for EPO to produce more EPO when the person is in hypoxic surroundings. This makes hypoxia-associated factor the new EPO; in low concentration it is equally effective and it cannot be traced as yet.

Hematocrit

Hematocrit, or Hct, is the percentage of red blood cells. The total amount of blood consists of about 45% red blood cells. The reference values are 41% to 55% for males and 36% to 48% for females.

Hct may be determined manually with the help of an Hct centrifuge. After the blood is centrifuged in a capillary tube, heavier red blood cells are at the bottom of the tube and the Hct value can be read. Hct is expressed in percentages.

There is also a formula to calculate Hct value.

$$\frac{\text{Mean cell volume} \times \text{number of red blood cells}}{1,000} = \text{Hct percentage}$$

The mean cell volume reference value is 83 to 98 mmol/l The red blood cell reference value is for males 4.2 to 5.5 $\times 10^{12}$ per liter and for females 3.8 to 5.0 $\times$ 1,012 per liter.

For example:

$$\frac{90 \times 5.0 = 450}{1,000 \quad 1,000} = 45$$

Hct in this example is 45%

Influences on Hct

Many different factors can influence the determined level of Hct.

- The method of determination adopted (There is a big difference between the "manually" determined Hct value and the calculated Hct value, with the calculated Hct value some 6% lower.)
- The laboratory (During repeated tests, we received totally different results from various laboratories that used the same method and the same blood sample, with a maximum of as much as 3 points difference.)

- Fluid intake (drinking)   Hct ↓
- Fluid loss (perspiration, diarrhea)   Hct ↑
- Hormonal regulation   Hct ↕
- Altitude   Hct ↑
- Anemia   Hct ↓
- Exogenous EPO   Hct ↑
- Various diseases   Hct ↑
- Alcohol use or abuse   Hct ↑
- Stress   Hct ↑
- Medication (diuretics)   Hct ↑
- Medication (minrin)   Hct ↓
- Infusion with a plasma replacement   Hct ↓
- Infusion with a sodium solution   Hct ↓
- Physical exercise   Hct ↑
- EPO   Hct ↑

When Hct increases it may indicate the use of exogenous EPO. However, an increase in Hct alone does not prove that exogenous EPO was used.

Under the influence of stress, Hct may show wide variations. During the stress of a race, plasma volume may decrease greatly, causing Hct to increase. The personal variation (i.e., day-to-day fluctuations) may be 10% to 12% in the same person. So Hct may be 48% on one day and 44% the next day.

Health Issues

There is no scientific evidence that an Hct value between 50% and 56% poses a risk for the athlete's health. With a high Hct the viscosity of the blood increases, but people living at high altitudes, who have very high Hct values, are not known for having more blocked or damaged blood vessels than those who live at low altitudes. There is absolutely no evidence that cyclists with an Hct between 50% and 56% run a higher health risk. Because nobody knows exactly what is a healthy and safe Hct value for an elite athlete, there is no scientific basis on which to ban an athlete from a race because of an increased Hct. For that reason alone, it is a ridiculous step to ban athletes with an Hct of more than 50%.

Normal Hct Values

Based on the normal values for men and women, some 10% to 15% of our healthy population has too high an Hct value. Based on the UCI principles, these people should be banned from intensive physical exercise because of their "abnormality."

Optimal Hct

Administration of EPO increases the oxygen transport capacity of the blood, so the blood carries more oxygen to the working muscles. If administration of EPO is not controlled sufficiently, Hct may increase too much. The increased viscosity of the blood then checks sufficient oxygen supply to the muscles, thus diminishing oxygen transport. Every athlete has an optimal Hct value, which is the value at which the muscles receive an optimum supply of oxygen. It is most likely that these values lie between 50% and 55% for most athletes. Hct values that surpass the optimum will reduce performance. Much scientific research remains to be done to answer the many questions about EPO and Hct.

Minrin

Minrin is a drug used for children who wet their beds. It may be bought as a nose spray, nose drops, pill, or injection liquid. The nose spray and injection liquid are preferable. Minrin contains desmopressine, which has a strong antidiuretic function that lasts 10 to 20 hours. Desmopressine retains blood in the vessels and thus minimizes urine production. If minrin is administered 2 hours before the UCI's morning Hct test and the athlete drinks a large amount of fluid, the Hct value may decrease by 2 to 3 full points. Minrin is not on the list of banned substances, but deliberately manipulating Hct is considered a doping crime by the International Olympic Committee.

Polycythemia Vera

In the disease polycythemia vera, also known as Morbus Vaquez-Osler, we see an unlimited increase of the number of red blood cells. This causes a higher viscosity and thus a higher Hct, which may explain most of the complaints. The cause of this disease is unknown. Its symptoms are fatigue, total malaise, and weakness, together with a deeply red face and dark red mucous membranes. The blood is very viscous. Even with the slightest effort the patient is dizzy and short of breath. The risk of thrombosis is enhanced.

Laboratory tests indicate the presence of this disease. Red blood cell count is often more than $10.0 \times 1,012$ per liter, with 4.2 to $5.5 \times 1,012$ per liter being normal. Hb is between 11.5 and 18.0 millimoles per liter with normal at 8.7

to 10.9 millimoles per liter. Hct is increased, often more than 60%, whereas normal is 41% to 55%.

In case of serious trouble, repeated bloodletting may help. It is interesting to note that the complaints and symptoms of this illness might, in theory, also be caused by excessive use of exogenous EPO.

Blood Values in Competition

The UCI uses Hct values as a basis for its health controls. The International Skiing Federation uses the Hb value. In fact, one method is no better or worse than the other, because there is a linear relationship between Hb and Hct (table 7.1). Determining both Hb and Hct does not provide a more accurate measure (figure 7.5, page 198).

Measuring Hct

Hct is measured in two ways, and the results are correlated but not identical.

Bayer Microspin M1101 Hct Meter

Many athletes use a Microspin to monitor their own Hct. The Microspin is a small, handy apparatus, but its results are 6% higher than those of the more advanced ADVIA-120.

Table 7.1 Relationship of Hb and Hct

Hb	Hct	Hb	Hct	Hb	Hct
2.0	12	7.2	35	12.4	59
2.1	13	7.3	36	12.5	59
2.2	13	7.4	36	12.6	59
2.3	14	7.5	37	12.7	60
2.4	14	7.6	37	12.8	60
2.5	14	7.7	38	12.9	61
2.6	15	7.8	38	13.0	61
2.7	15	7.9	39	13.1	62
2.8	16	8.0	39	13.2	62
2.9	16	8.1	39	13.3	63
3.0	17	8.2	40	13.4	63
3.1	17	8.3	40	13.5	63
3.2	18	8.4	41	13.6	64
3.3	18	8.5	41	13.7	64
3.4	18	8.6	42	13.8	65
3.5	19	8.7	42	13.9	65

Hb	Hct	Hb	Hct	Hb	Hct
3.6	19	8.8	43		
3.7	20	8.9	43		
3.8	20	9.0	43		
3.9	21	9.1	44		
4.0	21	9.2	44		
4.1	22	9.3	45		
4.2	22	9.4	45		
4.3	22	9.5	46		
4.4	23	9.6	46		
4.5	23	9.7	47		
4.6	24	9.8	47		
4.7	24	9.9	47		
4.8	25	10.0	48		
4.9	25	10.1	48		
5.0	26	10.2	49		
2.1	26	10.3	49		
5.2	26	10.4	50		
5.3	27	10.5	50		
5.4	27	10.6	51		
5.5	28	10.7	51		
5.6	28	10.8	51		
5.7	29	10.9	52		
5.8	29	11.0	52		
5.9	30	11.1	53		
6.0	30	11.2	53		
6.1	30	11.3	54		
6.2	31	11.4	54		
6.3	31	11.5	55		
6.4	32	11.6	55		
6.5	32	11.7	55		
6.6	33	11.8	56		
6.7	33	11.9	56		
6.8	34	12.0	57		
6.9	34	12.1	57		
7.0	35	12.2	58		
7.1	35	12.3	58		

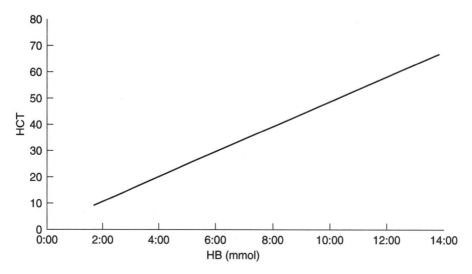

Figure 7.5 The linear relationship between Hct and Hb.

The Microspin centrifuges heparinized capillary tubes filled with blood. The centrifugation time and speed are standardized. The device is powered by batteries or an adapter. Filling the small capillary tubes requires some precision and skill, and they should be filled to the brim for reliable results. The scale on the glass is small, which might give rise to inaccurate reading; a small magnifying glass may help.

ADVIA-120

The ADVIA-120 is an advanced apparatus that is used in hospital laboratories to analyze blood. The UCI uses this apparatus for its morning Hct tests. There is a reliable correlation between the Hct values determined by the Microspin and the calculated Hct values of the ADVIA-120.

Correlation ($n = 14$): $y = -0.375 + 1.063 x$ (Hct in %), $r = 0.996$

So the results of the Microspin M1101 are about 6% higher than the ADVIA-120:

Hct% ADVIA-120 –6% = Hct% Microspin

An experienced analyst will achieve very high repeatability on both a high and a low Hct level. Table 7.2 shows data from two blood samples—one with a high Hct of 54% and the other with a low Hct of 28%, which were tested six times in two centrifuges.

Hct in Elite Athletes

On January 24, 1997, at a meeting in Geneva, in the presence of team leaders and prominent riders, the UCI decided to start preventive medical controls

Table 7.2   Sample Determinations

A	B
54	29
54	29
53	29
52	29
53	28

that consisted of Hct testing in the morning hours of the day of the race, with the objective to protect the health of the riders.

It was more than clear that these controls were meant to check the use of EPO. The regulations stipulated that those riders who were absent from the test, those who refused the test, and those whose Hct levels were more than 50% for males and 47% for females were to be banned from competition by means of a "declaration of incapability." The rider was admitted again when the next test, which at the earliest would be 15 days after the first test, reported an Hct lower than 50%.

If there is a reasonable indication that the rider has natural Hct levels more than 50% (for males) or 47% (for females), an extensive test protocol should be conducted. If it is verified that the rider indeed scores higher than the 50% line, he or she would obtain a UCI certificate permitting him or her to race with a natural Hct value over 50%. But this rider would be checked regularly by means of monthly blood sampling.

Although the UCI measures Hct values, the International Skiing Federation uses Hb. The standards followed by the International Skiing Federation are that in males, Hb should not exceed 18.5 grams per deciliter, or 11.49 millimoles per liter. Females' Hb should not exceed 16.5 grams per deciliter, or 10.25 (10.2 or 10.3) millimoles per liter.

The International Skiing Federation uses other standards than the UCI. For cyclists the Hct determination is a health measure, but there is little certainty about the health risks of a high Hct.

Hct More Than 50%

Between 1987 and 1996, Martin et al. (1997) found that Hct levels in 2.8% of 360 samples of Australian elite cyclists were greater than 50%. In a group of male and female Australian athletes, 3.4% had Hct values more than 50%. The Utrechts Medisch Centrum in the Netherlands investigated a group of elite athletes. In 5.9% of all athletes, the Hct value was greater than 50%. In athletes from high altitudes, that percentage was 20.5%; in the athletes from low altitudes, it was 0.8%.

Robin Parisotto, the scientist who developed the Australian antidoping test on EPO, found Hct values greater than 50% in 8 out of 151 blood samples, a percentage surpassing 5%. After the introduction of the health tests, a number of professional cyclists were excused because their natural Hct was greater than 50%; especially Colombians, who live the larger part of their life at altitudes of 3,000 to 4,000 meters, score high Hct values. When other sports also introduce Hct tests, it might turn out very difficult to stick to the limit. When the limit of 50% is maintained, a number of athletes will be banned unjustly.

In the Tour de France of 1984, the average Hct decreased from 45 to 42. In the Tour de France of 1988, the average was 43.5. In the Tour de France of 1997, the average had increased again to 45.5, probably due to the use of EPO.

Athletes from high elevations produce more natural EPO and therefore produce more red blood cells (table 7.3). Thanks to the higher Hb and Hct values of these athletes, they have a larger aerobic capacity than athletes from lower elevations, making them world-class athletes in endurance sports. It would be more "fair" if athletes surpassing the Hct 50% level would start in separate series. Tables 7.4 and 7.5 show typical Hct fluctuations in cyclists.

Using an Hct cutoff point of 50% for males and 47% for females cannot prove the use of EPO. Athletes from high altitudes, but some from low altitudes as well, run the risk of being unjustly banned from competition. In light of the facts, supported by literature, I believe that the Hct 50% rule cannot be maintained.

Table 7.3 Average Hct Values in Athletes From High Altitudes

Altitude (m)	Hct	Number	Country	Year
1,000	49.0	10	Colombia	1990
1,000	46.4	10	Colombia	1990 (runners)
2,600	49.3	10	Colombia	1990
2,600	47.9	10	Colombia	1990 (runners)
3,600	51.8	401	Bolivia	1988
3,600	53.6	8	Bolivia	1993
3,600	52.0	13	Bolivia	1995
3,700	52.2	29	Chili	1989
3,700	48.4	30	Nepal	1989
3,800	50.0	6	Bolivia	1992
3,900	53.3	13	Nepal	1979
3,950	62.0	6	Bolivia	1989

Table 7.4 Hct Fluctuations in a Cyclist Through the Years

Date	Hb	Hct	Red blood cells
Aug. 14, 1997	9.7	0.46	5.13
Mar. 23, 1998	10.4	0.52	5.62
June 29, 1998	9.7	0.48	5.21
Mar. 9, 1999	10.2	0.50	5.44
July 27, 1999	10.0	0.47	5.10
Jan. 24, 2000	10.9	0.52	5.59
Mar. 14, 2000	10.7	0.52	5.49
Apr. 27, 2000	10.4	0.50	5.40
May 2, 2000	10.5	0.51	5.40
May 9, 2000	10.1	0.49	5.22
May 18, 2000	9.8	0.47	5.04
May 29, 2000	10.4	0.50	5.40

Table 7.5 Hct Fluctuations in an Amateur Cyclist Through the Years

Ralf van Heugten	Hb	Hct	Red blood cells	Ferritin
Jan. 20, 1998	9.7	0.48	5.30	55
June 5, 1998	8.9	0.44	4.88	55
July 21, 1998	9.1	0.46	5.07	74
Feb. 23, 1999	10.3	0.50	5.53	72
May 20, 1999	9.2	0.46	5.01	66
June 24, 1999	8.9	0.47	5.12	69
July 22, 1999	9.2	0.45	4.97	82
Aug. 11, 1999	9.6	0.47	5.23	56
Apr. 6, 2000	9.7	0.47	5.12	96
May 9, 2000	9.1	0.44	4.80	109
Aug. 1, 2000	9.7	0.48	5.22	80

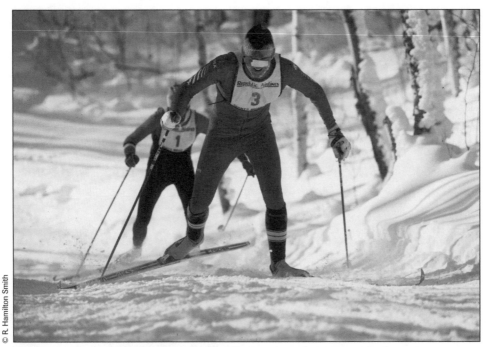

© R. Hamilton Smith

The International Skiing Federation uses Hb as a standard. Their limit values turn out higher than the Hct values used by the UCI.

Health and Hct Controls

At the January 24, 1997, meeting of the UCI, where it was decided to initiate blood tests with the objective of fighting the use of EPO, the following points were discussed:

Cycling has had a bad reputation for years because of the never-ending stream of stories about doping. EPO was particularly mentioned often as the miracle drug that could explain the supremacy of the Italian riders. By harshly fighting EPO use, cycling might return to a clean sport. The image improvement thus obtained might have a favorable effect on obtaining new sponsors. The sport might also become fair again, with equal chances for everybody. In addition, EPO use may endanger the health of the riders. The viscosity of the blood is increased by EPO use, which increases the risk of thrombosis and heart attack. The Hct value is a good standard for the blood's viscosity. Up till now the use of EPO could not be detected. A heightened Hct value is therefore an indirect method of measuring the likely use of EPO.

During the meeting, in the presence of team leaders and prominent riders, the UCI board decided unanimously to introduce blood and health tests. The objective was to protect the safety and health of the riders. It was decided that the blood's viscosity (i.e., Hct), should not exceed 50% for men and 47% for women. Hct controls were introduced to test this viscosity.

The UCI board stated that the blood tests that determine Hct should never be seen as doping tests but rather as preventive medical monitoring. A rider with an excessive Hct value would not be publicly seen as a doping culprit. The rider's license would be suspended for 15 days because participating in a race would be an unacceptable health risk.

It was decided that the Hct tests would be executed on the day of the race. Early in the morning, at 6 or 7 A.M., the riders would be awoken to be checked by UCI officials. In case of a Hct value exceeded 50% (men) or 47% (women), the rider would be forbidden to race for 15 days, and his or her license would be withdrawn. When in a second test, 15 days later, Hct was back to 50% or 47%, the rider would be found fit to race again and the license would be restored. Riders who could prove that their natural Hct value exceeds 50% or 47% could apply for dispensation; for example, this could be the case for Colombian riders who live and train at high altitudes at home, whose natural Hct often exceeds 50%.

But beside the Hct tests, done in the early morning hours, the UCI also introduced their health controls. In these checkups, the riders were systematically and extensively tested. In case of any anomaly, the rider's license could be suspended. According to the UCI these controls are meant to protect the riders' health.

When the UCI board introduced the Hct and health controls, the following ideas and arguments played a role:

- Cycling had a consistently bad doping image, caused by (among other factors) the endless stream of rumors about EPO.

- If EPO use could be limited the sport would become fair again, with equal chances for everybody.

- By introducing health controls not only do we protect the health of the riders, but doping abuse can be traced and fought. The call for health controls was strengthened by the rumor that in the Netherlands and Belgium alone, some 18 EPO deaths had occurred.

However, the introduction of a limit of 50% for men and 47% for women has not decreased the use of EPO. On the contrary; after the introduction of this limit, EPO use increased. The athlete's main concern turned to keeping below the 47% or 50% limit. Since that time, every professional cycling team has obtained its own Hct meter. So the measures have had an adverse effect, and the use of EPO has increased.

The safety and health argument is not convincing, and I believe it is a false argument. If the UCI really cared about the health of professional riders, the only solution would be to stop the sport of cycling as it is today. Professional cycling at elite level is per definition not good for anybody's health. Riding a Tour de France cannot be healthy for anybody: Three weeks at a stretch with extreme efforts every day; mountain rides with four to five slopes of the first category, in one day, in extreme weather conditions like tropical heat or harsh cold; the life-endangering descents and exhausting final sprints. In reality the UCI is not interested in the health of the riders. And they are right! Only the rider, the person, is responsible for his or her own health.

Health controls lead to nowhere; they are only very expensive. Not one athlete will benefit by them. Health controls unnecessarily medicalize sport and they are a stimulus for doping.

These controls were also introduced to polish the severely damaged image of cycling. Improving the image of cycling is indeed necessary if it is to survive at all, because the sport will die if sponsorship money cannot be raised, and sponsors do not wish to be associated with the negative image of doping. But the image improvement that was intended has not come about. The number of doping scandals has even increased since January 1, 1997. Just think of the Festina and TVM scandals of the Tour de France 1998, or the exclusion of Marco Pantani, 1 day before he was to win the Giro d'Italia of 1999. By October 2000, more than 60 professional riders had had their licenses suspended because of an excessive Hct value. This has generated an endless stream of negative publicity. In short, the effort to improve cycling's image has failed completely.

The argument that sports will be more fair with equal chances for everybody is invalid. Sport is not fair per definition, and it is the more interesting because participants with unequal qualities and backgrounds compete in the same event.

Following are some steps to take for a better doping policy:

- Clean the list of banned substances. The list should contain only those substances scientific evidence proves really enhance performance and endanger the athlete's health.
- Substances that cannot be traced should not be on the list.
- Athletes should be better informed—for example, through a medical or doping exam—before they get their licenses.
- The punishment should have a reasonable relationship with the seriousness of the event and should be in line with the punishment as in normal society.
- Doping victims should not be treated as criminals.
- Doping affairs should be dealt with by a civil judge instead of committees such as the UCI, and International Amateur Athletic Association (IAAF), and International Olympic Committee.
- Sports medical monitoring should receive the support it deserves. Sports doctors should never feel that they are on the brink of committing crimes and may be arrested at any time.
- Scientific research on doping and banned substances will have to be intensified. Subsidies and independent scientific research are required.
- Politicians should be mistrusted in doping matters.
- The public should be made to understand that doping use is not the same as drug abuse.

chapter 8

Nutrition

Those who exercise daily would be well advised to pay extra attention to everyday nutrition. More and more we see that well-balanced nutrition has a favorable effect on performance. Good nutrition, during the racing season and during the rest period, is essential.

The endurance athlete who practices good nutrition may improve performance by 7%. This improvement is seen in a lowered heart rate (HR) at equal loads. Therefore, this chapter covers all aspects of nutrition in relation to endurance sports.

Energy

Energy is required for all physical processes, both at rest and during activity. How much energy is required differs among people and may depend on age, sex, and physical activity. If energy intake is more than the required amount, it will be stored as a reserve in the form of fat, and body weight will increase. If energy intake is less than the required amount, the reserve of body fat will be used as a source of energy, and body weight will decrease. Thus, the amount of energy supplied by nutrition should equal the amount required for all physical processes.

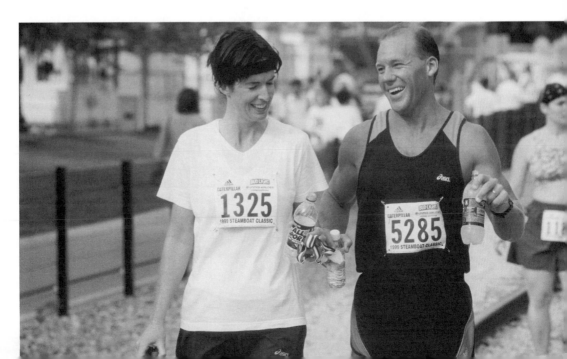

The amount of energy is expressed in kilocalories or kilojoules. Even at rest the body uses energy, and extra energy is needed for every activity. A normal energy requirement is about 2,000 to 3,000 kilocalories per day, although this varies depending on the person's daily activities. Exercise requires extra energy on top of the normal amount. The increase in energy expenditure depends greatly on the intensity and duration of physical exercise and the nature of the sport.

Carbohydrates and fats are energy-supplying nutrients. They are used within the body with the help of enzymes to provide an energy supply. The role of enzymes in energy supply is crucial. Enzymes only function in the presence of sufficient proteins, vitamins, minerals, and trace elements, so these must be present in the right quantities and composition. The food pyramid provides a good aid for making food choices.

Sources of Energy

The food pyramid shows all nutrients that should be present in everyday food. The pyramid is divided into four segments, each of which contains products belonging to one particular group. A good diet is composed of various foods in the right mix. Every food is a combination of various nutrients; there is no food that supplies all nutrients. In that sense, all foods are complementary to each other.

Good nutrition starts with good meals. These can be composed with the help of the nutrition pyramid. Each meal should contain one or more products out of every segment shown in figure 8.1. The athlete should choose a variety of foods from each segment.

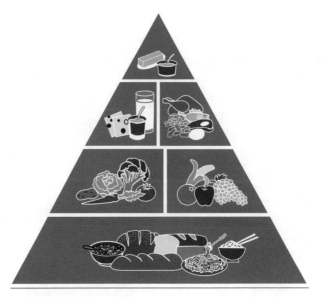

Figure 8.1   Food Guide Pyramid.

It is not simple to reach a well-balanced nutrition mix. Nearly all athletes eat too much fat and too few carbohydrates. During exercise the body uses both carbohydrates and fats, but carbohydrates are more important. Energy from carbohydrates can be used more quickly than energy from fats, and, more significant, the oxidation of carbohydrates consumes 16% less oxygen than the oxidation of fats. The body stores a small quantity of carbohydrates in the liver and muscles in the form of glycogen.

Carbohydrates

Carbohydrates are an important source of energy for many sports activities. Carbohydrates are capable of supplying more energy per time unit, compared with other nutrients. When the intensity of exercise decreases, the oxidation of fats begins to play a more important role.

A 400-meter runner gets his or her energy from the oxidation of carbohydrates. For a cyclist or marathon runner, sports in which endurance is more important, the oxidation of fats will be more important. A cyclist in the final sprint or in an escape from the pack will have to shift to carbohydrate oxidation again because fats do not cover all energy needs. In cycling, the role of the "domestiques" (cyclists who help the leading cyclist) is based on this principle. The domestique provides a windbreak for the leader, enabling the leader to spare carbohydrate reserves for the final spurt. The domestique is burning carbohydrates and by the end of the race is burned out.

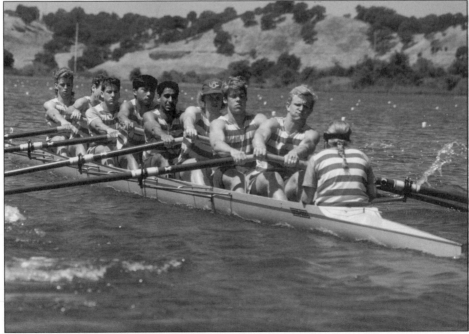

© Mary E. Messenger

The amount of extra calories required for maximum effort depends largely on age, sex, and sport.

The store of carbohydrates in trained persons is about 700 to 800 grams. This store is sufficient to maintain a submaximal effort during 60 to 90 minutes. If these carbohydrates are not reloaded in the 60- to 90-minute effort, glucose content of the blood will decrease. That is the moment when the athlete feels exhausted. When carbohydrates are used up, fats and proteins take over as main sources of energy. This change in energy source inevitably decreases performance.

Fats

Western diets generally contain too much fat. Most athletes have fat reserves of 10 to 15 kg. Theoretically this amount is enough for 15,000 minutes of walking or 4,000 minutes of marathon running. Recreational runners who want to lose weight (i.e., burn fat reserves) should exercise at low intensities for maximal fat oxidation.

As mentioned previously, intensive effort requires carbohydrate (CHO) oxidation and less intensive effort requires fat oxidation. Training makes it possible to shift from carbohydrate to fat oxidation, so that after a training period maximum performance capacity increases. A well-trained athlete is capable of performing up to 80% of his or her maximum effort by using fats as a source of energy. When the athlete performs between 80% and 100% of maximum capacity, energy will be supplied out of carbohydrates. Untrained persons use fat oxidation for about 50% of their maximum performance levels, so they have to change to carbohydrate oxidation sooner.

After a period of training, a shift takes place in the direction of more fat oxidation, which means that the well-trained athlete burns fats longer and therefore can save carbohydrate reserves. Schematically, this shift is represented in graph 139.

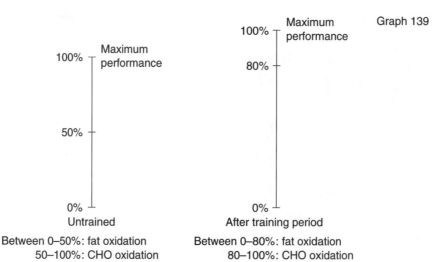

Graph 139

Proteins

Until a few years ago, people believed that proteins had no role in energy supply during exercise. Recent investigations have proven that proteins do play a role. In endurance sports, 5% to 15% of energy comes from proteins. This percentage may even be higher when there is a succession of heavy workouts or when the duration and intensity of workouts increase even more, such as marathons and triathlons.

It is not favorable for the athlete to get a large share of energy supply from proteins, because the proteins that are used come partially from the muscles. The muscles are somewhat consumed, which can have a negative effect on performance. The current recommendation is that an endurance athlete needs 1.5 to 2 grams of proteins per kilogram of body weight per day. So an endurance athlete of 70 kilograms needs $70 \times 1.5 = 105$ grams to $70 \times 2 = 140$ grams of protein per day. Milk proteins are preferable, because they contain all essential amino acids in considerable amounts, are easy to digest, and can easily be concentrated.

Oxidation of Carbohydrates, Fats, and Proteins

The oxidation of carbohydrates, fats, and proteins supplies different amounts of energy. Burning 1 gram of carbohydrates yields 17.1 kilojoules (4.1 kilocalories), 1 gram of fat yields 39.6 kilojoules (9.5 kilocalories), and 1 gram of protein yields 23.7 kilojoules (5.7 kilocalories).

At first glance fat seems to supply most energy. Yet this is not always true, because these three fuels require different amounts of oxygen. In intensive exercise, the amount of oxygen that reaches the muscle per time unit is more important than the amount of fuel present in the muscle. In other words, oxygen supply is the limiting factor.

When the body is burning carbohydrates, 1 liter of oxygen yields 21.1 kilojoules (5 kilocalories); when burning proteins, 1 liter of oxygen yields 18.7 kilojoules (4.5 kilocalories); and when burning fats, 1 liter of oxygen yields 19.8 kilojoules (4.7 kilocalories). So the oxidation of carbohydrates supplies more energy per liter of oxygen. During exercise the body will automatically use the fuel that supplies the most energy with the given intake of oxygen. Therefore, the body will use fats for exercise of low intensity because more energy is supplied out of 1 gram of fat and because oxygen is not a limiting factor at this low level.

When the exercise is more intensive, oxygen intake does become a problem. In these cases the carbohydrates, which give more energy per liter of oxygen, are preferred. Proteins follow a long route in the body before they are available as a source of energy. Therefore, they are not the most economical fuel despite the favorable fuel/oxygen/energy ratio.

Oxygen needs of carbohydrates, fats, proteins, and alcohol

Carbohydrate oxidation:	1 gram, 17.1 kilojoules	1 liter oxygen, 21.1 kilojoules
Fat oxidation:	1 gram, 39.6 kilojoules	1 liter oxygen, 19.8 kilojoules
Protein oxidation:	1 gram, 23.7 kilojoules	1 liter oxygen, 18.7 kilojoules

Because carbohydrates need relatively less oxygen, they are used in intensive exercise. Fats require more oxygen, so less intensive exercise uses fat. Proteins follow a long, energy-consuming route.

Basic energy expenditure can be determined by using table 8.1. The table assumes that the person sleeps 8 hours per day, using 1.0 kilocalorie per kilogram of body weight per hour of sleep. The table also assumes that the person performs 16 hours of light work per day (e.g., office work or teaching) or normal household work that requires an average of 1.5 kilocalories per kilogram of body weight per hour.

Basic energy expenditure of a person who weighs 75 kilograms is calculated as follows:

Energy use during 8 hours of sleep = 75 × 8 × 1 = 600 kilocalories

Energy use during 16 hours of light work = 75 × 16 × 1.5 = 1,800 kilocalories

Thus, basic energy use per 24 hours is 2,400 kilocalories.

Table 8.1 Basic Energy Consumption Depending on Body Weight

Body weight (kg)	Energy consumption (kcal per 24h)
50	1,600
55	1,760
60	1,920
65	2,080
70	2,240
75	2,400
80	2,560
85	2,720
90	2,880
95	3,040
100	3,200

Total Energy Expenditure

Total energy expenditure is the sum of basic energy use and sports energy.

Total energy = basic energy + sports energy

Energy use for various sports and at various intensities is shown in the sports energy figure 8.2. If table 8.1 gives 10 kilocalories per hour of exercise, 8.5 kilocalories per hour of activity is added to basic energy.

Energy expenditure during sports activities

Example 1

This example gives energy use during a 2-hour endurance run, at a pace of 10 kilometers per hour, for a runner weighing 70 kilograms. Table 8.2 shows that 10 kilocalories will be consumed per hour. The net energy expenditure of the sports activity itself is 10 – 1.5 = 8.5 kilocalories per kilograms per hour. The basic energy expenditure is deduced from the total.

This 70-kilogram runner uses 70 × 2 × 8.5 = 1,190 kilocalories for the 2-hour endurance run. The runner's basic energy expenditure is 2,240 kilocalories, and the total energy expenditure per day is then 3,430 kilocalories.

Example 2

This example gives the energy use of a cyclist during an intensive ride with some strenuous climbs.

Duration of the workout: 6 hours

Body weight of the cyclist: 65 kilograms

Sports energy table (table 8.2): 17.5 kilocalories per kilogram per hour

Net energy expenditure: 17.5 – 1.5 = 16 kilocalories per kilogram per hour

Energy expenditure during ride: 16 3 65 3 6 = 6,240 kilocalories

Basic energy expenditure: 2,080 kilocalories

Total energy expenditure: 8,320 kilocalories

Example 3

Marathon runner

Body weight: 65 kilograms

Marathon time: 02:30:00

Pace: 16.8 kilometers per hour

Sports energy table (table 8.2): 19.5 kilocalories per kilogram per hour

Sport energy measurement

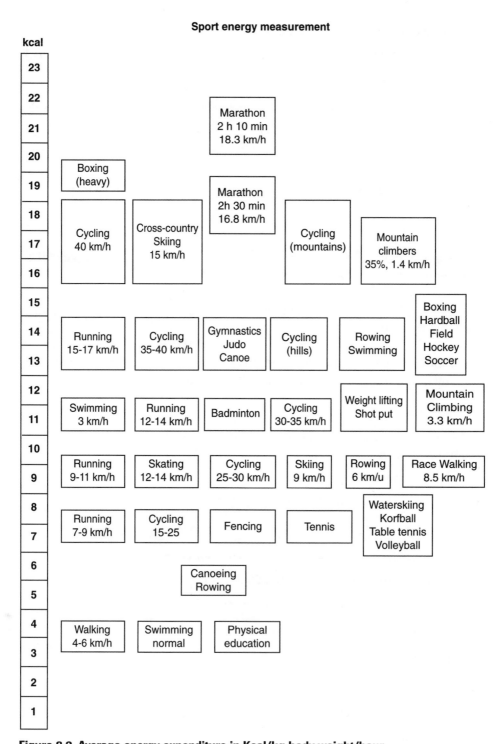

Figure 8.2 Average energy expenditure in Kcal/kg body weight/hour.

Net expenditure: 19.5 – 1.5 = 18 kilocalories per kilogram per hour

Energy expenditure for the marathon: 18 3 65 3 2.5 = 2,925

Basic energy expenditure: 2,080 kilocalories

Total energy expenditure: 5,005 kilocalories

Table 8.2　Sports Energy Expenditure

Example 1: 2 h cycling 25-30km/h, net: 10-1.5 = 8.5 cal/km/hr, + base energy: Total energy per day:

50	55	60	65	70	75	80	85	90	95	100
850	935	1020	1105	1190	1275	1360	1445	1530	1615	1700
1600	1760	1920	2080	2240	2400	2560	2720	2880	3040	3200
2450	2695	2940	3185	3430	3675	3920	4165	4410	4655	4900

Example 2: 1.5 h judo, canoeing, or soccer: net: 14.5-1.5=13 cal/km/h: + base energy: Total energy per day:

50	55	60	65	70	75	80	85	90	95	100
975	1072.5	1170	1267.5	1365	1462.5	1560	1658	1755	1853	1950
1600	1760	1920	2080	2240	2400	2560	2720	2880	3040	3200
2575	2832.5	3090	3347.5	3605	3862.5	4120	4378	4635	4893	5150

Example 3: 5 h cycling 40 km/h w/ intermittent climbing: net: 17.5-1.5 = 16 cal/km/h: + base energy/: Total energy per day:

50	55	60	65	70	75	80	85
4000	4400	4800	5200	5600	6000	6400	6800

Cyclists at this level will weigh approximately 60-80 kg.

Nutrition for Endurance Sports

During exercise, although dependent on the athlete's condition and the intensity of exercise, carbohydrates are the most important fuel for the resynthesis of adenosine triphosphate (ATP). Per liter of oxygen intake, carbohydrates form 16% more ATP than fats. A well-trained athlete performs a triathlon at an intensity of 60% to 70% of his or her $\dot{V}O_2$max . At this level of intensity, both fats and carbohydrates are used as fuels. The lower the intensity of exercise, the larger the share of fat oxidation for energy supply. Because muscles burn both carbohydrates and fats, more carbohydrates are used as the intensity of exercise increases.

The Carbohydrate Reserves

Under normal conditions, the amount of glycogen in the liver and muscles is 400 to 500 grams. One kilogram of carbohydrates supplies about 4,000 kilocalories. So the carbohydrate store in the body supplies 1,600 to 2,000 kilocalories. The glycogen store within the muscles is the fuel for muscular activity. Normally this store is enough for 60 to 90 minutes of submaximal exercise. The speed at which muscle glycogen is consumed depends on the level of intensity. The more intensive the exercise, the sooner the glycogen store will be exhausted. Graph 140 shows how glycogen is exhausted during 90 minutes of exercise.

When the glycogen store is exhausted, a low blood glucose content will occur, which results in a feeling of being totally "worn out." Other important symptoms of low blood glucose content are decreased performance, hunger, clammy and sweaty feeling, weak and powerless legs, and lightheadedness. Also the nervous system does not function well, and movement is uncoordinated (think of athletes who reach the finish swaying and crawling). By consuming adequate carbohydrates, the athlete may avoid exhausting the glycogen reserve.

Various Types of Carbohydrates

Carbohydrates consist of simple sugars and complex sugars. The simple sugars or monosaccharides are glucose and fructose, which can be taken up by the blood directly without further digestion. For quick replenishment during or after a race, glucose and fructose solutions are most suitable. The complex sugars are disaccharides and polysaccharides. Disaccharides are sucrose and maltose; polysaccharides are starches and glycogen.

The complex sugars are broken down to small particles (glucose) by the digestive enzymes. Only then is uptake into the blood possible. Because this digestive process takes some time, the complex sugars are taken up more slowly. During long-duration exercise, a combination of simple and complex

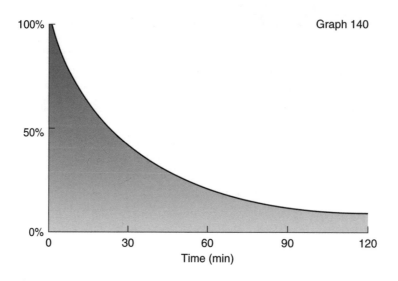

Graph 140

sugars is advisable. The slow and rapid uptake of these two kinds of sugars guarantees a constant supply of carbohydrates to the blood.

Glucose is stored in the liver and muscles in the form of glycogen. So there are two kinds of carbohydrates present in the body: the glucose in the blood and the glycogen in muscle tissue and the liver. A regulatory mechanism influenced by the hormones glucagon and insulin ensures that the glucose content of the blood is fairly constant. A high glucose content of the blood, as occurs immediately after a meal, stimulates insulin secretion. With the help of insulin, glucose is stored as glycogen in the liver and muscles.

The glycogen in the liver keeps glucose content of the blood constant. This is important because the nervous system can only use glucose as a fuel and therefore depends on the glucose present in the blood. The glycogen in the muscles is used as a fuel for muscular activity. Figure 8.3 shows different types of sugars.

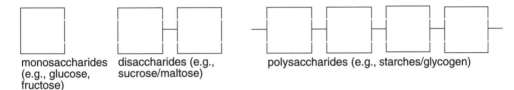

monosaccharides (e.g., glucose, fructose) disaccharides (e.g., sucrose/maltose) polysaccharides (e.g., starches/glycogen)

Figure 8.3 Types of sugars.

The Banana

The banana is a compact unit of carbohydrates and energy. One banana has an average weight of 150 grams and contains 32 grams of carbohydrates, the superfuel for intensive endurance sports. The fruit is rich in magnesium (50% more than potatoes), potassium, and vitamin C and—like the potato—starches. Starch consists of long chains of glucose molecules, which during digestion, are broken down into glucose molecules. Moreover, the banana contains small amounts of free sugars such as glucose, fructose, and saccharose (which is known as beet or cane sugar). Bananas taste good and because of the high moisture content are easy to eat with a dry mouth during prolonged exercise. Furthermore, this fruit contains indigestible fibers, which reach the colon as bulky

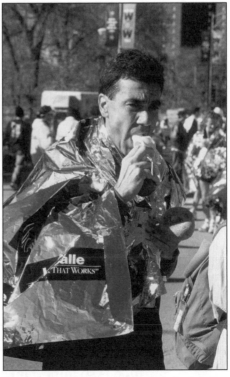

Bananas act as superfuel to replenish lost energy stores.

substance. This will increase feces volume and consistency, which helps prevent diarrhea.

The degree of digestibility depends greatly on the ripeness of the banana. The banana has its own process of ripening in which the starch structure slowly changes from indigestible to very digestible. In this ripening process, the content of free, rapid-absorption sugars increases. Unripe bananas (yellow with green tips) land in the colon 75% undigested. Ripe bananas (yellow with black spots on the peel) are digested nearly completely and taken up by the blood, a detail of major importance to endurance athletes. When unripe bananas are eaten, gas will be formed and the indigestible bulk will result in gastrointestinal complaints and the urge to defecate.

Foods rich in carbohydrates

Bread	Molasses	Fruit juices
Currant bread	Honey	Gingerbread
Raisin bread	Raisins	Candies
Cookies	Currants	Muesli bars
Pastry	Dates	Glucose
Potatoes	Figs	Cereals
Rice	Peas	Carbohydrate drinks
Macaroni	Onions	Jam
Spaghetti	Broad beans	Sweet drinks
Fried rice	Marrowfat peas	Sugar
Fried noodles	Fruit in syrup	Banana

The Fat Reserve

A well-trained athlete with a body weight of 75 kilograms and a fat percentage of 10% has a fat reserve of 7.5 kilograms. Body fat contains about 7,000 kilocalories per kilogram, so in total this athlete has about 50,000 kilocalories stored in the form of fats. Practically spoken, there is always a sufficient amount of stored fat.

Energy Consumption for Events

Because nutrition is so important to athletic success, athletes must plan for proper nutrition before, during, and after an endurance event. Two of the most demanding endurance events that require optimal nutrition are the long triathlon and the marathon.

The long triathlon consists of swimming (3.8 kilometers), cycling (180 kilometers), and running (42.2 kilometers). In well-trained triathletes, intensity during the whole triathlon is about 60% to 70% of their $\dot{V}O_2$max. The most elite athletes may even reach about 80% of their $\dot{V}O_2$max, whereas less well-trained people (those who require 15 hours for the event) may reach about 40%.

A trained athlete with a body weight of about 75 kilograms will expend about 10,000 kilocalories during the long triathlon, 50% of which will be supplied by fats and 50% by carbohydrates. The fat reserve is more than enough to supply these 5,000 kilocalories. However, the carbohydrate reserves are always insufficient for the long triathlon, because the maximum carbohydrate reserve is about 2,000 kilocalories. To cover the total energy need, some 3,000 kilocalories must be consumed in the form of food, which means an intake of 750 grams of carbohydrates. This simple sum shows that at the end of the long triathlon, the complete glycogen reserves are exhausted, demonstraiting a decreased blood glucose content and lowered performance capacity. To avoid this, the triathlete will have to consume even more energy, beyond the 3,000 kilocalories. Exhaustion of the glycogen reserve may be avoided by taking in 2,000 kilocalories more in the form of carbohydrates. So the total carbohydrate intake should be 5,000 kilocalories or 1,250 grams. An example of this can be seen in Figure 8.4 and table 8.3.

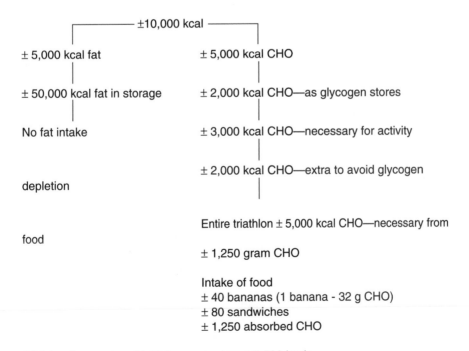

Athlete who requires 14-15 hours requires ± 7,500 kcals.

Figure 8.4   Energy consumption of top triathletes.

Table 8.3	Holland Triathlon										
Total energy (kcal)	Total time (h)	Swimming			Cycling			Running		
		(km/h)	(h)	(kcal)	(km/h)	(h)	(kcal)	(km/h)	(h)	(kcal)
Winner 10,620	9	4.0	1.0	1,275	40.0	4.5	5,670	13.0	3.5	3,675
15 hours 7,410	15	2.0	2.0	1,200	22.5	8.0	3,360	8.5	5.0	2,850

In a marathon, the intensity is higher than in a triathlon. Elite and well-trained athletes run a marathon at 75% to 90% of their $\dot{V}O_2$max. Because intensity of exercise is higher, the share of carbohydrate oxidation will increase strongly. With every increase of intensity, carbohydrates are used more and fats are used less as the fuel for energy supply. If an athlete does not consume carbohydrates during the marathon, the reserves will be depleted after 60 to 90 minutes, resulting in low blood glucose levels and a lower performance level. The pace cannot be maintained then, because the body will switch from carbohydrate to fat oxidation. The low blood glucose content makes the athlete feel hungry, clammy, sweaty, and weak.

The moment of glycogen depletion is generally around 30 to 35 kilometers. This depletion can be avoided by consuming small amounts of carbohydrates during the run, far before the 30th kilometer. It also makes sense to load extra carbohydrates by eating meals rich in carbohydrates for some days before a long endurance effort. This postpones the moment of depletion.

Nutrition Before an Endurance Effort

The meals taken before long endurance efforts should be rich in carbohydrates. This carbohydrate-rich diet should be started some days before the race to fill glycogen depots as much as possible. This method of carbohydrate loading is called overcompensation. There are various methods of overcompensation.

With the first method, during the last 3 or 4 days before the race, the normal varied diet changes into a carbohydrate-rich diet. The glycogen supply within the muscles now increases from 15 to 25 grams per kilogram of muscle tissue. During these 3 or 4 days, there are no more vigorous workouts.

The second method consists of a combination of nutrition and physical work. First, the reserves are depleted in a long workout. Then, a few days of carbohydrate-rich nutrition follow. Glycogen reserves may be doubled by this method, rising from 15 to 30 grams per kilogram of muscle tissue. Again, there are no vigorous workouts on the days of the carb-loading diet.

The third method is also based on physical exercise and nutrition. Again the glycogen reserves are fully depleted by means of exhausting workouts, but now 3 days of a carbohydrate-limited diet follow. These days nutrition may contain many fats and proteins. There may even be a few strenuous workouts to further deplete the reserves. Then 3 days of a carbohydrate-rich diet follow without vigorous workouts. The glycogen reserves may now increase from 15 to 50 grams per kilogram of muscle tissue.

Under normal conditions, glycogen reserves are 350 grams. With these various nutritional manipulations, glycogen reserves may increase to 800 grams.

The third method is difficult. A 1-week regime requires a lot of self-discipline. After the exhausting workouts, 3 days of a diet rich in fats and proteins follow. During these days the athlete will feel very tired, which is a psychological disadvantage just before an important race. Another disadvantage of an extreme carb-loading diet is an increased amount of water in the muscles, causing a weight gain. With a maximal carb-loading diet, this gain may be 2 to 4 kilograms, which can cause a feeling of heaviness and muscle stiffness. Diarrhea also occurs when one is not used to carbohydrate-rich nutrition. The carb-loading methods 1 and 2 are easier in the preparatory phase. Graph 141 compares the results of the three methods.

Nutrition Immediately Before a Race

The last small meal before a long race should be consumed 2 hours before the race, at the latest; bigger meals should be consumed at least 3 hours before.

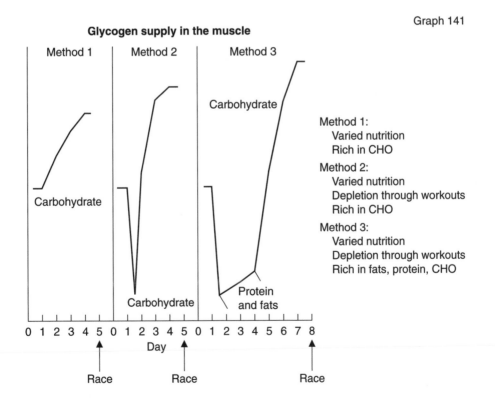

Graph 141

Glycogen supply in the muscle

Method 1:
  Varied nutrition
  Rich in CHO

Method 2:
  Varied nutrition
  Depletion through workouts
  Rich in CHO

Method 3:
  Varied nutrition
  Depletion through workouts
  Rich in fats, protein, CHO

These meals should contain many carbohydrates, so that the glucose content of the blood remains constant and the athlete performs well during the effort.

Because the body uses some energy and water after the last meal, it is advisable to drink a sugar solution of 300 to 500 milliliters some 5 minutes before the race begins. This will give the athlete a higher blood glucose content at the start. However, using large amounts of glucose or sugar, especially in liquid form, less than 1 hour before the start is not advised.

The Insulin Shock

If the athlete consumes 75 grams of glucose in 300 milliliters of water 45 minutes before the race starts, the pancreas will produce extra insulin. Insulin ensures that glucose from the blood is stored in the muscles. Thus, at the start of the effort, insulin levels will be higher than normal. Through this combination of exercise and heightened insulin level, blood glucose content will decrease too fast and the result will be a more rapid exhaustion during exercise. This unfavorable phenomenon is called an insulin shock.

By not consuming food 2 hours before exercise or high amounts of sugar 1 hour before exercise, the athlete avoids this phenomenon because insulin will not be produced during exercise. Graphs 142 and 143 illustrate insulin shock.

For this reason, the sugar concentration in sports drinks should not exceed 2.5 grams of glucose per 100 milliliters of water. This drink may be taken in till half an hour before the start without a negative influence on performance. Diluted fruit and vegetable juices may also be taken in till half an hour before the start.

Liquid Nutrition Before the Race

Many athletes suffer from digestive trouble before races because of nervousness. These complaints, such as diarrhea, nausea, vomiting, and abdominal

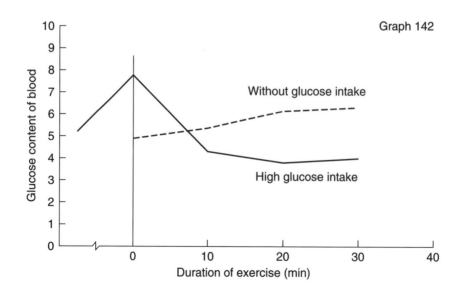

Graph 142

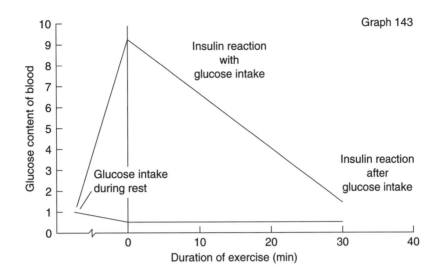

Graph 143

cramps, may harm performance considerably. They might be avoided by replacing solid food with liquid food. Liquid food has a well-balanced nutritional value, tastes good, is easy to digest, and passes through the stomach quickly.

Because the food is liquid, water is also consumed together with energy, so liquid food may be the solution for athletes with nervous abdominal complaints. The body requires some time to get used to any new nutritional regime, so the athlete should experiment with a liquid diet long before the racing season.

Methods to Delay Glycogen Expenditure

The last meal before the event should be rich in fats and proteins and poor in carbohydrates: eggs, cheese, meat, and yogurt, but few or no sweets. This selection results in a higher fat content and a relatively lower sugar content in the blood before the start of the exercise. This combination stimulates the muscles to burn more fats, and glycogen expenditure will be delayed. This method is best for efforts of long duration in which the pace, especially at the start of the race, will not be too high. This dietary regime should also be tried long before the race.

Caffeine improves endurance performance because it stimulates the breakdown of fats and thus saves the glycogen reserves. This method works best for those who normally consume no caffeine. Sometimes caffeine may have adverse effects such as stomach complaints, heart palpitations, sleeplessness, and nervousness. Caffeine pills, which contain the same amount of caffeine as one cup of coffee, work considerably better, probably because the caffeine from pills is taken up better than the caffeine from a beverage. If the athlete uses caffeine, endurance runs at an intensity of 91% maximal HR, or

Table 8.4

Product	Quantity	Caffeine in mg
Cup of coffee	240 ml	100
Cup of tea	240 ml	50
Glass of Coca-Cola	350 ml	40
Cup of caffeine-free coffee	240 ml	10
Glass of chocolate milk	350 ml	15-40
Chocolate bar (pure)	30 gr	10
Chocolate bar (milk)	30 gr	25
APC	one pill	60

85% $\dot{V}O_2$max, may be maintained for 23-85% longer. Table 8.4 lists the caffeine content of various substances.

Caffeine is on the doping list. The athlete will be found positive if more than 12 micrograms of caffeine is found per milliliter of urine. It is impossible to know exactly how many cups of coffee or other beverage may be drunk within this limit. This differs from person to person and also depends on factors such as environmental temperature and the degree of dehydration. A dehydrated athlete will produce concentrated urine at the doping check and therefore will be found positive at lower levels of caffeine consumption.

The athlete should experiment with the effects of coffee in workouts long before the event and can start by drinking a caffeinated beverage 1 hour before the workout. This amount can be increased to a certain reasonable point, but five cups of strong coffee within 1 hour before the race puts the athlete at risk of having a positive test for doping. Coffee in combination with painkillers containing caffeine is even more risky.

Although caffeine is known to improve endurance performance, there is no evidence that coffee has any positive effect on marathons. However, an intake of 300 milligrams of caffeine (three cups of strong coffee) may result in a time gain on distances up to 10,000 meters. Also, caffeine intake may lengthen the duration of a heavy workout by some 20%.

Nutrition During an Event

Exercise longer than 60 to 90 minutes exhausts glycogen reserves. It is important to avoid this by eating regularly and thus replenishing any glycogen shortage before glycogen exhaustion occurs. During physical exercise, the gastrointestinal channel functions less because most of the blood goes to the working muscles. The food passage in the bowels is also slower. This is the reason why many people cannot handle food during exercise. When the level of exercise is not too high, solid food may be taken such as cookies, raisins, bread, bananas, and candies. As an alternative, when solid food is not tolerated any more, carbohydrate drinks can be consumed. The concentration of these drinks should not be too high: Glucose content should not be more than 2.5 grams per 100 milliliters of water. If the concentration is higher, the stomach will empty more slowly, delaying the absorption by the blood.

During races the athlete should regularly take small portions of solid or liquid food, although eating during exertion should always be trained before a race. The gastrointestinal channel is very trainable in the digestion of food during exercise. During a long effort, the replenishment of carbohydrates and fluid is essential. Carbohydrate intake during exercise saves muscle glycogen reserves and avoids low blood glucose content. This makes the athlete feel fit and delays fatigue (graphs 144 and 145).

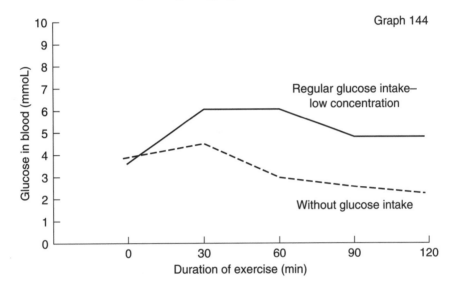

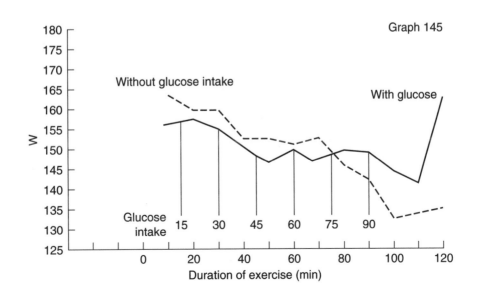

Nutrition After Exercise

After a heavy endurance workout, the rapid replenishment of fluid, minerals, and electrolytes is a necessity. A rapid replenishment of the energy reserve is also essential, the more so when another heavy workout is planned for the next day.

Within a few minutes after the finish, the athlete should consume liquid sugars or a high-energy drink, even if he or she doesn't feel hungry. From 1 hour after the race onward, it is possible to have a substantial solid meal rich in carbohydrates. If another race is due the next day, this meal should contain foods that are easy to digest, such as cream and butter (fats); bread, jellies, and rice (carbohydrates); fish, soft-boiled egg, cheese, and dairy products (proteins); and fresh fruit and fruit juices.

Important Nutrition Rules
for Endurance Athletes

- Do not experiment with a new nutrition pattern just before a race. Test new nutrition patterns long before the event. The gastrointestinal channel can be trained to digest food during exercise.
- Eat and drink regularly during exercise. If you start eating or drinking at the moment of hunger or thirst, you are too late.
- Ensure full glycogen reserves for endurance exercise longer than 60 to 90 minutes.
- The last meal before a race or workout should be eaten 2 to 3 hours before.
- The biggest mistake is drinking too little.
- Glycogen reserves are depleted after 60 to 90 minutes of submaximal performance.
- Liquid food passes through the stomach faster than solid food.
- A carbohydrate-loading diet may double the carbohydrate reserves.
- Consuming large amounts of glucose or sugar, especially in liquid form, less than 1 hour before the race is inadvisable.
- Liquid sugars consumed immediately after an endurance effort enhance recovery.

Fluid and Endurance Sports

The biggest mistake an athlete can make during exercise is drinking too little. Fluid loss during long endurance workouts decreases circulating blood volume. The blood then becomes thicker and more viscous. To keep oxygen supply at a constant level, HR increases. No fluid intake during exercise results in a distinctly higher HR in comparison with adequate fluid intake. In other words, if the athlete drinks too late or too little or does not drink at all, performance inevitably will suffer and exhaustion will occur sooner.

A good fluid balance during exercise is of major importance. More than 60% of the body consists of water. This water has several important functions including the solution and transportation of numerous substances, heat regulation, and excretion of toxic substances with sweat and urine.

During physical exercise a lot of heat is produced, causing body temperature to rise. To avoid overheating, the body will start perspiring, which costs the athlete much fluid loss. During strenuous exercise in hot weather, sweat loss may be as high as 3 liters per hour. If this loss is not compensated, performance capacity will decrease. Even a slight loss of 2% of body weight may impair performance. With a loss of 3% to 6% of the body weight, strength and endurance capacity will decrease by about 30%. An athlete weighing 70 kilograms will not be able to maintain his or her performance level with a fluid loss of 3 to 4 kilograms (i.e., 4% to 6% of body weight). With a fluid loss of more than 6% of body weight, the consequences may be enormous (see table 8.5, page 226).

Well-trained people lose less water and salt during exercise than untrained people. Through exercise, the body learns how to sweat more efficiently. To determine the amount of fluid loss during exercise under varying conditions (training, races, heat, cold, etc.), the athlete should weigh before and after exercise. The difference is a good estimation of fluid loss. If an athlete loses 3 kilograms in one workout, the workout has not been very efficient. Such a workout does more harm than good.

Weight loss during physical exercise is not entirely due to dehydration. It is known that glycogen may bind to quite an amount of water. When these glycogen reserves are depleted, some water is lost that does not contribute to dehydration. Especially when the athlete has followed a carb-loading diet, body weight may increase by 2 to 3 kilograms due to water bound to glycogen. So some weight loss during long-duration exercise is acceptable.

There is a golden rule for drinking: Drink regularly during exercise and do not wait until you are thirsty. When you start drinking when you are thirsty you are too late. Thirst is felt when fluid loss is already 2% to 3%. In general, athletes drink too little during exercise. Only 30% to 50% of sweat loss during exercise can be compensated by drinking.

The osmolality of a drink is the major factor that decides if a drink passes through the stomach rapidly enough to be absorbed by the body. Osmolality indicates the number of diluted particles, consisting of carbohydrates, salts, and minerals, compared with the number of particles in the blood. Drinks may be hypotone, isotone, or hypertone in comparison with blood.

Hypotone: The drink contains fewer particles than blood.

Isotone: The number of particles equals the number in the blood.

Hypertone: The drink contains more particles than the blood.

Water does not contain any of these particles, which is why water passes through the stomach quickly. But drinking water during prolonged intensive exercise may cause some problems. The taste is not agreeable, which will not induce the athlete to drink regularly. This is a disadvantage, because the feeling of thirst is suppressed during exercise. After water, the hypotone drinks pass the stomach most rapidly. Hypertone drinks pass slowly because they are diluted first in the stomach, and this may cause a full and sloshing feeling in the belly (see table 8.5).

Because the salts and carbohydrates lost during physical exercise should be compensated for, the ideal thirst quencher is a hypotone drink. This drink contains small amounts of carbohydrates and minerals. Suitable drinks during exercise are diluted fruit juices and hypotone thirst quenchers. However, drinking too much hypotone fluid can result in a serious disturbance of the electrolytes called water intoxication. During exercise shorter than 1.5 hours, water is sufficient (preferably mineral water rather than tap water). Many sports drinks are too concentrated, which results in a slower stomach passage. Gastric complaints such as nausea, a sloshing stomach, a full feeling, and vomiting may result.

Table 8.5 Fluid Loss and Performance

Fluid loss in percentage of body weight	Results
2	Disturbed heat regulation, body temperature rises, thirst
3	Less endurance capacity
4–6	No resolve to eat and drink, headaches, decreased strength
6–10	Overheating, muscle cramps, nausea, shortness of breath, fatigue, vomiting
>10	Difficulty swallowing, fluid intake only possible via infusion, fainting, coma, death

Fluid rules for endurance athletes

- The liquid should be hypotone.
- The drink should contain a maximum of 2.5 to 4 grams of glucose or fructose per 100 milliliters of water.

- The liquid should be cool: 4 to 12 degrees Celsius (40 to 55 degrees Fahrenheit).
- The taste should be agreeable.
- Thirty minutes before the race or workout, the athlete should drink 400 to 600 milliliters of water or hypotone drink.
- During the race, the athlete should drink 100 to 200 milliliters of hypotone drink every 15 to 20 minutes. For cyclists the rule is one bottle every hour.
- After the race, the athlete should eat food that is a little more salty than normal and should drink mineral solutions to compensate for the electrolytes lost during exercise (sodium, potassium).
- Performance distinctly increases when the athlete drinks regularly during activities that last longer than 60 minutes.

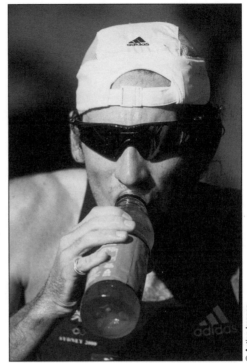

© Action Images

Good hydration is the key to strong performance.

Depending on the amount of fluid loss, the athlete should drink 100 to 200 milliliters every 15 to 20 minutes. The weather conditions and the intensity of exercise strongly influence fluid loss and therefore the need for fluid replenishment. The stomach tolerates the passage of about 800 milliliters of fluid per hour maximally. When the intake is more, some problems may arise such as a full and sloshing feeling. On a hot day in the Tour de France, when the riders have to ride a stage of 200 kilometers or more, a fluid intake of 10 to 15 liters per person per day is no exception.

About 30 minutes before the start of the exercise, about 400 to 600 milliliters of a carbohydrate drink can be taken. If the exercise is shorter than 1 hour, these extra carbohydrates are not necessary; fluid regulation, rather than absolute fluid intake, is the important factor. In a certain sense, a hypotone drink can certainly compensate for fluid loss. During exercise longer than 1 hour, a drink with carbohydrates can be taken in a "quiet" phase of the race or workout. It takes some time, however, before this is absorbed by the blood.

chapter 9

Heart Rate Patterns

Training analyses as well as the research literature show that athletes often train at the wrong intensities. This chapter discusses heart rate (HR) patterns from many different athletes and many different sports and activities. First the chapter analyzes a number of endurance workouts.

Lactate Determination

Lactate determination has become an essential element of coaching. After lactate levels are determined, the exact methods and intensities of training can be assessed. Analyses of workouts show that many athletes train incorrectly.

Cyclo-Cross

Table 9.1 shows two lactate determinations (L1 and L2) at two different time points during a group workout of 13 cyclo-crossers. There was no fixed training task. It was an average workout that was done two to three times a week at the same intensity.

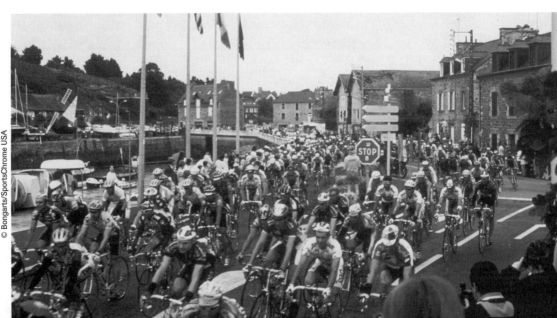

© Bongarts/SportsChrome USA

Table 9.1	Lactate Determination (mmol/l) of 13 Cyclo-Crossers												
Participants													
	1	**2**	**3**	**4**	**5**	**6**	**7**	**8**	**9**	**10**	**11**	**12**	**13**
L 1	8.2	5.0	4.3	4.2	15.7	11.1	8.9	4.1	3.9	7.2	7.2	12.5	8.5
L 2	8.7				14.3	9.8	10.7			4.8	4.8	12.1	12.6

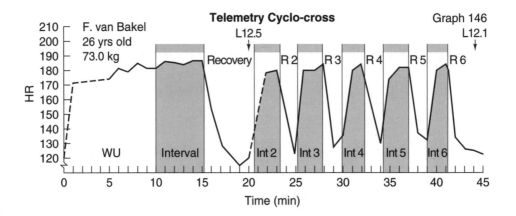

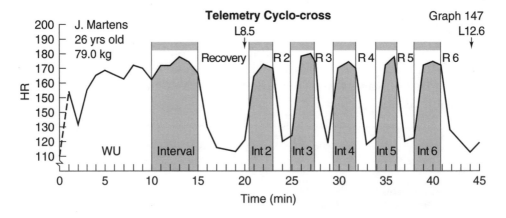

The HR curves of participants 12 and 13 (see graphs 146 and 147) were made up telemetrically.

The lactate values varied widely for the 13 participants. This means that the effect of this workout differed between participants. Participants 2, 3, 4, 8, and 9 trained aerobic capacity. The other participants reached high lactate values, which means that their lactate tolerance was trained but not their aerobic capacity. Three workouts of this kind per week, plus races on the weekends, make a training load that is far too heavy.

Maximum performance capacity inevitably will suffer from this training load. The high lactate values decrease aerobic endurance. Because of this heavy training method, many cyclo-crossers show a distinct decline in achievement during the season. It is quite a job to convince athletes to change this approach by limiting the number of workouts with high lactate values. These workouts must be replaced by workouts that train aerobic endurance, in which lactate levels do not exceed 6 millimoles per liter.

Many athletes are not satisfied when they do not feel totally "worn out" after a workout; they believe workouts must result in the same feeling of fatigue that follows races. This fatigue is brought about by high lactate values. By just changing the training mix, performance capacity may be maintained or—at least for some athletes—even increased considerably.

Swimming Workouts

During sprint workouts, the creatine phosphate (CP) system is trained. High lactate values during a sprint workout are undesirable, because the formation of lactate indicates the use of the anaerobic system. Lactate values during sprint workouts should not surpass 6 to 7 millimoles per liter. Table 9.2 shows data for five swimmers who participated in a sprint workout of about 16 seconds of maximum effort, followed by about 16 seconds of recovery. Total workout time was about 30 minutes.

Again, distinct differences in lactate values are seen in exactly the same workout. The data for Participant 2 are especially noteworthy. By taking longer recovery pauses or by reducing the length of the sprints, an athlete could avoid reaching such high lactate values. Only then will the workout be a real sprint workout. Participants 1, 3, 4, and 5 reached the right lactate values, which indicates that their workouts went according to plan.

Table 9.3 shows the data for 13 swimmers who undertook workouts of 30 seconds of maximum effort, followed by 15 seconds of recovery. Lactate values for this group workout show large differences, even though all participants had the same training task. A large percentage of the participants did not achieve a sprint workout but rather a lactate tolerance work-

Table 9.2 Lactate Determination (mmol/l) of 5 Swimmers After Sprint Workout					
Participants					
	1	**2**	**3**	**4**	**5**
L 10 min	5.9	14.0			
L 20 min	7.0	14.0			
L 30 min	6.4	14.6	5.8	4.3	5.6

Table 9.3	Lactate Determination (mmol/l) of 13 Swimmers After 30 Seconds, Maximum Effort											
Participants												
1	**2**	**3**	**4**	**5**	**6**	**7**	**8**	**9**	**10**	**11**	**12**	**13**
L 7.0	7.2	4.1	12.0	6.3	6.6	7.8	5.1	4.0	5.5	11.9	10.1	6.7

out. The training task did not work well for them, because they simply lacked the feeling for the right training intensity.

After a 15-minute warm-up, five swimmers performed a 30-minute endurance workout, with the results shown in table 9.4. The participants were accustomed to the intensity of this endurance workout. Lactate was determined after 15 and 30 minutes of endurance work (L1 and L2). Then a recovery pause of 20 minutes followed and after that an interval workout of 12×60 meters at 80% of maximum intensity. Halfway through and at the end of the interval workout, lactate was determined again (L3 and L4).

Only Swimmer 4 performed well according to the task and achieved the correct intensity for an endurance workout. The training impulse was excellent for optimal use of the aerobic energy-supplying system. Also the interval part went well for Participant 4. The lactate values were high enough, which means that the anaerobic system was taxed sufficiently. For Participants 1, 2, 3, and 5, neither the endurance part nor the interval part was effective. The tasks were not carried out well by these swimmers, because an optimal endurance workout takes place in the lactate range of 2 to 4 millimoles per liter, and the lactate tolerance workout should fall between 6 and 10 millimoles per liter.

Table 9.4	Lactate Determination (mmol/l) of 5 Swimmers After Endurance Workout				
Participants					
	1	**2**	**3**	**4**	**5**
L 1	3.3	1.7	1.6	4.9	2.7
L 2	2.4	1.8	1.6	4.3	1.4
L 3	1.0	1.3	4.9	8.4	1.8
L 4	1.2	1.0	2.9	8.8	1.4

Cycling Workouts

Table 9.5 shows data for a cycling workout with three participants on a hilly road (Berg en Dal near Nijmegen, The Netherlands). Four laps were done at maximum intensity. At the end of every lap, the last part of which was a 2.5-kilometer climb, lactate was determined. HR was measured throughout the workout (see graphs 148, 149, and 150).

For every participant, the workout was an ideal lactate tolerance workout; that is, the anaerobic system was trained. As an aerobic endurance workout, it was too intensive. This type of workout once a week is enough. In a period of many races it is even superfluous, because in that case the races are the ideal means to train lactate tolerance.

Table 9.5	Lactate Determination (mmol/l) of 3 Cyclists at Maximum Intensity			
	Participants			
	1	**2**	**3**	
L 1	9.1	9.1	7.6	1st lap
L 2	7.0	8.6	7.3	2nd lap
L 3	3.7	5.1	8.2	3rd lap
L 4	5.6	4.8	12.0	4th lap

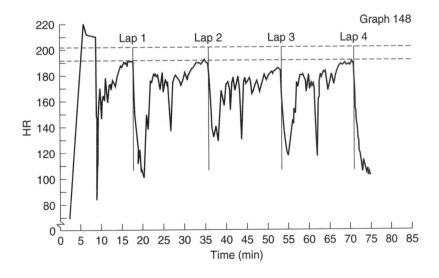

Graph 148

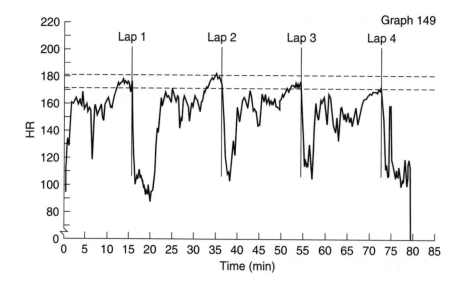

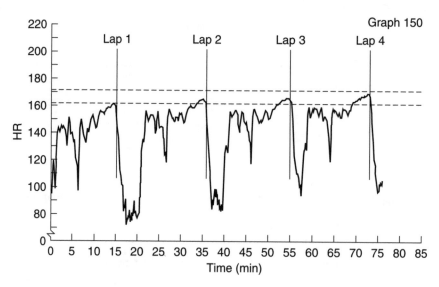

Long-Distance Running

After a 20-minute warm-up, 15 long-distance runners did an endurance workout of 30 minutes, with the results shown in table 9.6. A recovery period of 15 minutes was followed by an interval workout. The endurance workout and the intervals were done at the usual intensity. The first lactate determination was after 15 minutes of endurance work (L1) and the second after 30 minutes (L2). L3 was determined halfway through the intervals and L4 at the end of the workout.

Table 9.6 Lactate Determination (mmol/l) of 15 Runners After an Endurance Workout

| | \multicolumn{15}{c}{Participants} | | | | | | | | | | | | | |
	1	2	3	4	5	6	7	8	9	10	11	12	13	14	15
L1	2.3	1.5	1.1	2.6	0.8	0.8	1.0	1.5	1.1	2.2	1.7	5.1	4.5	1.3	1.0
L2	1.3	1.4	0.9	1.8	0.8	0.6	0.9	1.4	0.8	2.5	1.9	5.1	4.2	1.4	0.9
L3	0.8	2.9	7.3	6.4	8.3	4.1	10.1	10.0	9.9	8.0	5.8	11.1	5.7	8.6	4.4
L4	0.8	2.9	5.8	7.2	9.7	8.4	8.5	12.3	7.7	10.1	6.8	9.9	6.9	9.4	5.2

The training stimulus of an endurance workout is right when it results in lactate values between 2 and 4 millimoles per liter. For 12 out of these 15 runners, the intensity was too low for an endurance workout. Only Runners 10, 12, and 13 ran at the right intensity. The light acidosis of Runner 12 probably had no negative effect. Exceeding the 4 millimoles per liter limit slightly during endurance workouts is not too serious. It would be ideal to determine this runner's HR deflection point (HRdefl) exactly to be sure of the right intensities.

The interval workout, which trains the lactate system, requires values between 6 and 10 millimoles per liter. For most runners this part of the workout went better. But again there were some who did not achieve the training task. Graph 151-165 show HR curves for the 15 runners in the test.

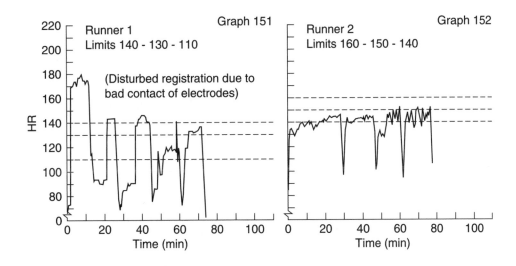

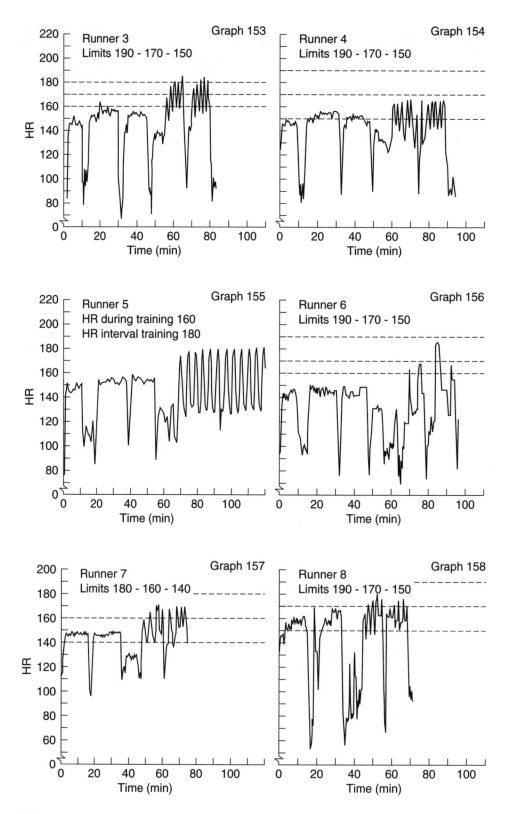

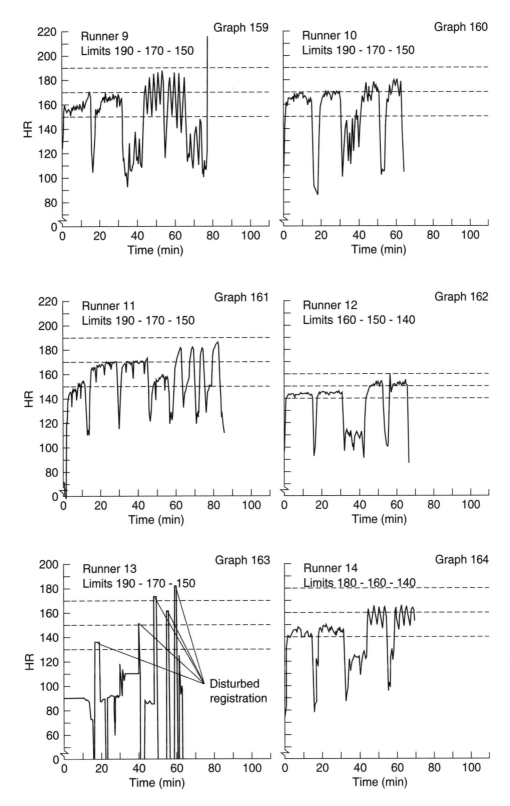

237

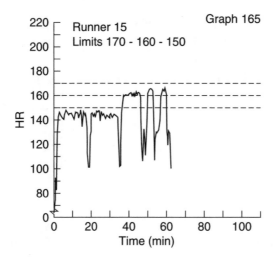

Graph 165

Lactate determinations were done in three long-distance runners (see table 9.7), and an HR record was made for two of them (graphs 166 and 167). The task was to perform an endurance run at the usual intensity. L1 was determined after 15 minutes and L2 after 30 minutes, that is, at the end of the workout. There is no HR curve for Runner 1.

Runner 1 had a good endurance workout at the right intensity. Runners 2 and 3 did not carry out the training task correctly, and they performed a lactate tolerance workout rather than an aerobic endurance workout.

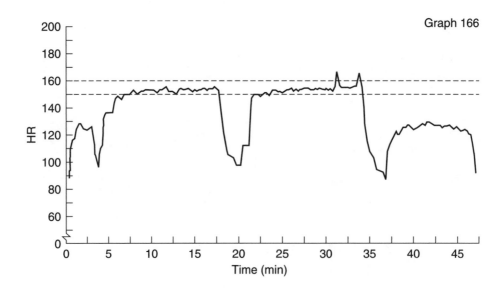

Graph 166

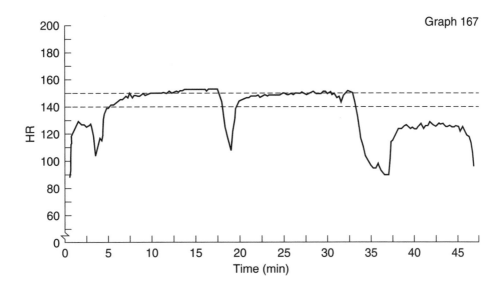

Graph 167

Table 9.7   **Lactate Determination (mmol/l) of 3 Long-Distance Runners**

	Participants		
	1	**2**	**3**
L 1	4.0	7.5	9.5
L 2	4.1	9.1	10.9

European Football

Football players were given the task of performing six uphill runs at maximum pace; their lactate curves are shown in graph 168. When HR had decreased to 120, there was another start.

During this type of workout, maximum lactate values are reached between 15 and 24 millimoles per liter. These high lactate values require a minimal recovery time of 48 hours. During this period, the risk of injuries is very high, and technical skills cannot be trained, because coordination is disturbed. This type of workout is typical of football. Unfortunately, it decreases endurance capacity and should be eliminated during the preparatory period.

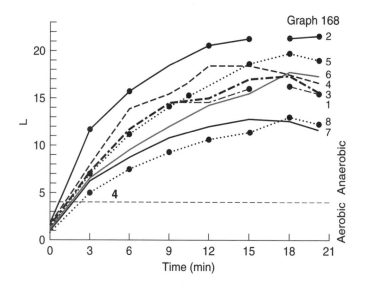

To investigate whether a football player performed vigorously during a match, HR and lactate content were determined. It appeared that the HR of top football players was higher than 85% of their maximum for the greater part of the match.

HR patterns of pro football players in Sweden showed that the average oxygen consumption during a normal match is about 80% of their maximal oxygen consumption ($\dot{V}O_2$max). This means that the football player should have an excellent aerobic endurance capacity and a football-specific anaerobic endurance capacity. Graph 169 shows that the football player has to handle lactate values between 4 and 14 millimoles per liter during the match. Exercise during a football match is often anaerobic, with all its unfavorable consequences such as disturbed coordination and a higher risk of injuries.

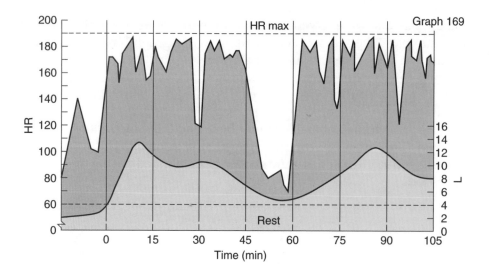

A 17-Year-Old Sprinter

Graph 170 and table 9.8 provide data from a workout for a 17-year-old sprinter that consisted of three series: 5× 60 meters, 5× 60 meters, and 5× 70 meters. Lactate after warm-up was 4.3 millimoles per liter. Lactate after 3 minutes of easy running was 2.9 millimoles per liter (onset lactate). HR at the onset of the second and third series was remarkably high.

This young sprinter performed three to four of these workouts per week. In the previous year he had not improved, and the number of injuries had increased greatly. This workout resulted in very high lactate values and might be seen as a highly intensive lactate tolerance workout. As a sprint workout it was a complete failure. One such a workout per week was probably too much; three to four of these workouts would certainly cause problems. This workout diminished the athlete's performance and caused numerous injuries.

During sprint workouts, lactate levels must not increase too much; this can be avoided by taking longer recovery periods. In that recovery time, the complete phosphate battery (CP and adenosine triphosphate) can be recharged.

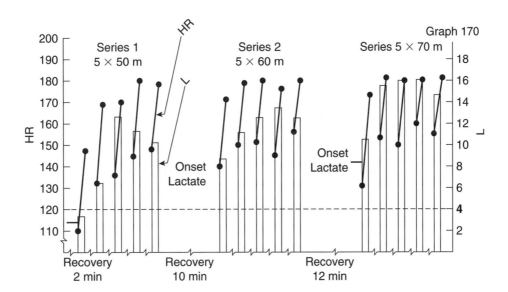

Table 9.8 Sprint Workout for a 17-Year-Old

	First series			Onset lactate 2.9 (mmol/l)	
Meters	HR	HR	Time (sec)	Recovery (min)	Lactate (mmol/l)
1st 50	110 > 147		5.8	2	3.7
2nd 50	132 > 168		5.9	2	6.3
3rd 50	136 > 169		5.9	2	12.8
4th 50	145 > 179		6.0	2	11.2
5th 50	145 > 178		6.0	2	10.2

After this series, 10 min of easy running

	Second series			Onset lactate 7.1 (mmol/l)	
Meters	HR	HR	Time (sec)	Recovery (min)	Lactate (mmol/l)
1st 60	140 > 172		6.8	2	8.6
2nd 60	150 > 179		7.0	2	11.1
3rd 60	151 > 180		7.3	2	12.6
4th 60	145 > 176		6.9	2	13.5
5th 60	157 > 180		6.9	2	12.7

After this series, 12 min of easy running

	Third series			Onset lactate 8.3 (mmol/l)	
Meters	HR	HR	Time (sec)	Recovery (min)	Lactate (mmol/l)
1st 70	132 > 174		8.2	2	10.6
2nd 70	154 > 181		8.0	2	15.5
3rd 70	151 > 180		8.3	2	16.1
4th 70	161 > 181		8.4	2	16.2
5th 70	156 > 181		8.4	2	14.8

Comparisons of Performance Capacity

The practical examples discussed in this book show how training programs can be improved. But lactate determination also provides other important information; for example, performance capacity can be assessed exactly. Questions like, "Am I good enough for a certain category?" or "What time can I achieve in my present condition?" can be answered. When performance capacity is known, athletes can be compared. Undoubtedly, in the future, selection procedures will be based on lactate determinations.

Performance capacity is assessed in a condition test, the quality of which determines whether performance capacity is judged accurately. One of the first requirements for a valid condition test is that the athlete is tested during normal exercise: the swimmer in water, the runner on the road or track, and the cyclist on his or her bike or an ergometer. Testing a swimmer on a treadmill or ergometer provides an inaccurate measure of swimming capacity. Thus, the lactate curve should be determined sport specifically if we are to learn the athlete's sport-specific capabilities.

Sport-specific capability may be defined as the pace that can be reached at lactate 4 (L4), also called the V4 pace. This V4 pace is an important indicator of real performance capacity. An improved V4 pace always is accompanied by an improvement of maximum performance capacity. Based on the V4 pace, the athlete's race times can be predicted. Regular determinations of the V4 pace show the athlete's condition. (See table 9.9).

Table 9.9 Male and Female Swimmers—V4 Pace

V4 m/sec Level	100 m Females	100 m Males	200 m Females	200 m Males	400 m Females	400 m Males
National	1.331	1.440	1.281	1.304	1.177	1.343
European	1.467	1.565	1.412	1.478	1.264	1.480
World	1.553	1.634	1.473	1.531	1.438	1.532

Note: The average sport specific endurance capacity on various distances. The higher the level, the higher V4 pace.

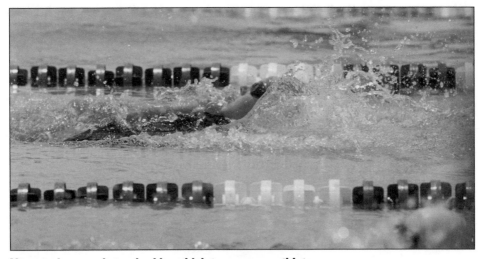

V4 pace is a good standard by which to compare athletes.

Swimmers

A certain level requires a certain V4 pace. If this demand is not met, the results will be disappointing.

Part of this section was taken, with permission, from a publication by Geert and Piet Leinders, sports medical doctors at Merelbeke, Belgium.

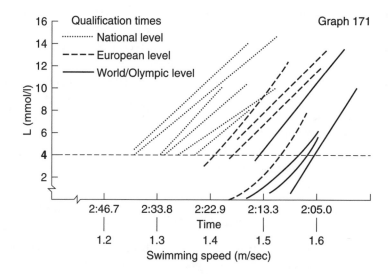

Cyclists

If cyclists of different categories are compared, you see a progressive improvement of achievements at 2 millimoles per liter and 4 millimoles per liter (the aerobic and anaerobic thresholds). From the novice to the junior, to the amateur, to the professional, the lactate curve gradually shifts to the right (graph 171).

If we compare cyclists of the same category, we see clear differences among them (table 9.10).

It is understandable that pro cyclists, examined in the same period of the season, have the same condition. The difference in their lactate values is probably based on different talents. In table 9.11, P1 is a successful pro cyclist who is 26 years old. P2 and P3 are new in professional cycling. As expected, P2 has already had some remarkable successes. P4 is the classic example of the "domestique," the helper of the leading cyclist; he has made perfect use of his limited talents during his professional career. P3, the less talented newcomer, overestimated his possibilities and was dismissed by a large cycling team, which had contracted him the year before. Clearly, performance capacity in cyclists is shown by their lactate curves.

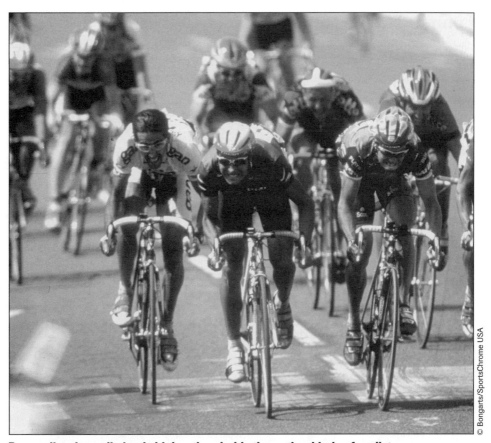

Pro-cyclists have distinctly higher thresholds than other kinds of cyclists.

Table 9.10 Comparison of Four Levels of Cyclist

	Novice 15-16 years	Junior 17-18 years	Amateur	Professional
W at 2 mmol/L	200	270	320	360
W at 4 mmol/L	270	315	376	425

Table 9.11 Comparison of Four Pro Cyclists

4 pro cyclists	P1	P2	P3	P4
W at 2 mmol/L	360	345	320	320
W at 4 mmol/L	425	394	380	371

Long-Distance Runners

Actual running times were compared with laboratory tests at 4 millimoles per liter. Table 9.12 shows data for 13 athletes in order of their achievement in the laboratory at 4 millimoles per liter (kilometers per hour and HR on a treadmill). Tables 9.13, 9.14, and 9.15 compare the athletes' best times in races and the laboratory tests at 4 millimoles per liter.

It is remarkable that the same order is nearly always reached and that racing results correlate perfectly with the test results at 4 millimoles per liter. According to Mader (1978), achievement at the anaerobic threshold is the best criterion for judging an athlete's aerobic capacity. The figures in these tables bear evidence to that statement.

Table 9.12 Long-Distance Runners

Order	Name	Achievement at 4 mmol/L	
		km/h	HR
1	G.W.	21.2	179
2	M.D.	21.2	185
3	V.M.	21.0	176
4	D.E.	20.7	175
5	B.H.	19.8	177
6	D.S.E.	19.8	189
7	D.G.	19.7	176
8	M.G.	18.6	168
9	L.J.M.	18.0	176
10	V.L.	17.8	170
11	P.R.	17.75	185
12	E.A.	17.6	164
13	G.L.	15.8	178

Table 9.13 Aerobic Endurance of Short Duration (2-8 Min)

Name	Running time	Order in the 4 mmol/L test
1,500 m		
1. G.W.	03:40.02	1
2. V.M.	03:45.16	3
3,000 m		
1. G.W.	07:55	1
2. D.S.E.	08:22	6
3. B.H.	08:24	5
4. D.E.	08:30	4
5. D.G.	08:32	7
6. V.L.	09:10	10
7. E.A.	09:40	12

Table 9.14 Aerobic Endurance of Medium Duration (up to 15 Min)

Name	Time (min:sec)	Order
5,000 m		
1. G.W.	13:55.28	1
2. M.D.	14:14.03	2
3. V.M.	14:23	3
4. D.E.	14:30	4
5. D.S.E.	14:39	6
6. B.H.	14:43	5
7. D.G.	14:52	7
8. V.L.	15:42	10
9. E.A.	17:02	12

Table 9.15 Aerobic Endurance of Long Duration (longer than 15 minutes)

Name	Time (min:sec)	Order
10,000 m		
1. G.W.	00:29:40	1
2. M.D.	00:29:43	2
3. D.E.	00:30:13	4
4. B.H.	00:30:38	5
5. D.S.E.	00:30:55	6
6. D.G.	00:31:37	7
7. V.L.	00:32:40	10
8. E.A.	00:35:02	12
Semi-marathon Race of 21 km 750 m		
1. M.D.	01:9:24	2
2. M.G.	01: 9:32	7
3. L.J.M.	01:9:40	9
4. G.L.	01:13:02	13
5. P.R.	01:13:30	11

Four Distance Runners

Lactate results were recorded for four distance runners at different times, as shown in tables 9.16 through 9.19. Tests were administered on January 17, April 15, May 6, July 25, September 3, September 5, and November 26.

Table 9.16 Distance Runner 1—Examined January 17 and July 25

	January 17 (km/h)	July 25 (km/h)
Aerobic threshold (2 mmol/L)	18.6; HR 170	17.1; HR 163
Anaerobic threshold (4 mmol/L)	21.2; HR 183	19.3; HR 178

Table 9.17 Distance Runner 2—Examined September 5 and May 6

	September 5 (km/h)	May 6 (km/h)
Aerobic threshold (2 mmol/L)	18.0; HR 150	17.8; HR 155
Anaerobic threshold (4 mmol/L)	19.8; HR 175	19.7; HR 172

Table 9.18 Distance Runner 3—Examined November 26 and April 15

	November 26 (km/h)	April 15 (km/h)
Aerobic threshold (2 mmol/L)	17.3; HR 155	18.5; HR 165
Anaerobic threshold (4 mmol/L)	20.0; HR 171	21.2; HR 180

Table 9.19 Distance Runner 4—Examined September 3 and July 25

	September 3 (km/h)	July 25 (km/h)
Aerobic threshold (2 mmol/L)	16.2; HR 160	17.2; HR 160
Anaerobic threshold (4 mmol/L)	18.5; HR 177	19.2; HR 177

Lactate curves for the four runners are shown in graphs 172 through 179. In graphs 172 and 173, the lactate curve has the same pattern, but performance both at the aerobic and at the anaerobic threshold decreased after the first test. This deterioration can be explained by an injury, which forced the athlete to temporarily diminish his training program in both volume and intensity.

In graphs 174 and 175, the second runner's performances at 2 and 4 millimoles per liter were practically identical. Lactate curves were the same from 2 millimoles per liter onward. Less than 2 millimoles per liter, the curve of May 6 is clearly more favorable.

The athlete depicted in graphs 176 and 177 showed a distinct improvement in all aspects of his endurance capacity. This resulted in a remarkable progress as a distance runner and excellent racing results. He even became Belgian champion on one distance.

The distance runner depicted in graphs 178 and 179 also showed a considerable improvement of his test results. It is remarkable that he scored

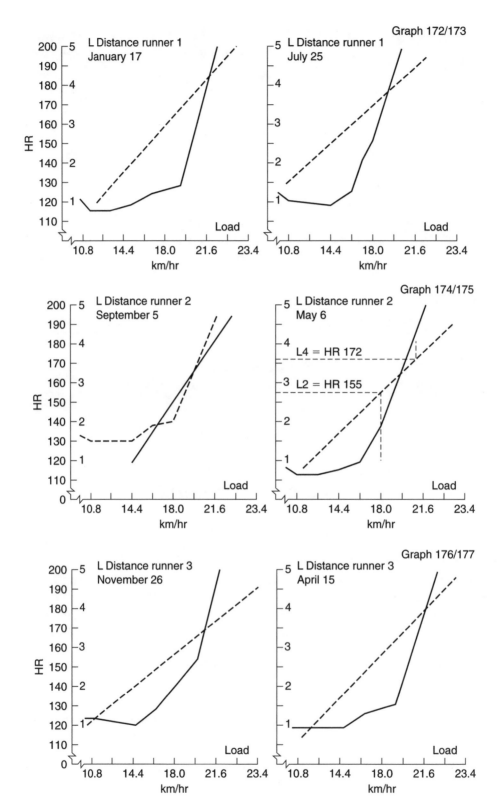

Graph 172/173

L Distance runner 1
January 17

L Distance runner 1
July 25

Graph 174/175

L Distance runner 2
September 5

L Distance runner 2
May 6

L4 = HR 172

L2 = HR 155

Graph 176/177

L Distance runner 3
November 26

L Distance runner 3
April 15

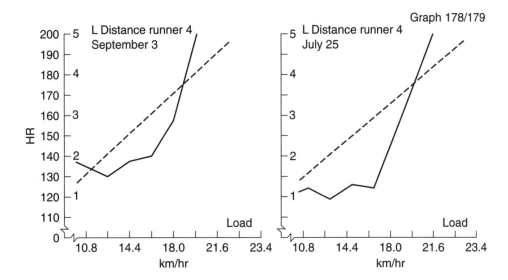

Graph 178/179

the same HRs at 2 and 4 millimoles per liter on the two test dates. His pace, however, was practically 1 kilometer per hour faster.

This comparison of distance runners at different time points clearly shows the possibility of correctly evaluating an athlete's condition.

Heart Rate Patterns of Various Workouts

With the help of constant HR recording, the athlete's workout can be analyzed objectively to determine whether the athlete has carried out the training task correctly. Training mistakes, if any, can be corrected based on this evaluation. In this way an athlete learns exactly what the correct intensities feel like. Assessing and readjusting workouts are the most important uses of an HR monitor with a memory bank.

The curve in graph 180 represents a recovery workout.

Test details

L4 = HR 175

L2 = HR 160

During a recovery workout, lactate levels must never exceed 2 millimoles per liter. Well-trained athletes often perform their recovery workouts far below 2 millimoles per liter. For the athlete depicted in graph 180, it is well known that his workouts are often too intensive. He cannot easily keep himself in check. Because of these overly intensive workouts, his racing results are often disappointing.

The task for this workout was keeping HR under 150. In that way lactate content would not rise over 2 millimoles per liter. If the athlete's HR during

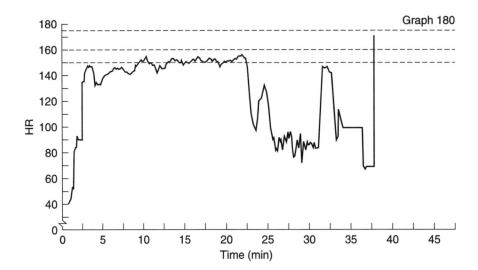

the workout exceeded 150, the HR monitor beeped to warn the athlete to slow down. Because the workout was stored in the memory bank, it could be analyzed and discussed afterward.

The curve in graph 181a represents an intensive endurance workout on the road by a cyclist. The data of this rider were recorded in a bicycle ergometer test in the laboratory.

Test details

L4 = HR 164
L3 = HR 157

An intensive endurance workout for a well-trained cyclist is in the lactate range between 3 and 4 millimoles per liter. During this workout, the cyclist's HR permanently fluctuated around 160, so this workout may be considered an intensive form of endurance training. The task was to ride at maximum and constant speed for 1 hour. The dips in the curve are traffic situations that temporarily disturbed the constant speed.

Graph 181b is an example of an intensive endurance workout by a marathon runner. The task was to run units of 10 minutes at an HR between 140 and 145. After such a period, about 10 minutes was allowed for recovery. This runner had the following values:

Test details

L4 = HR 144
L3 = HR 138

The intensive parts were run at an HR between 140 and 145. The training task was carried out excellently.

The curve of graph 182 represents a workout by a cyclist on a bicycle ergometer. It is an example of intensive repetitions.

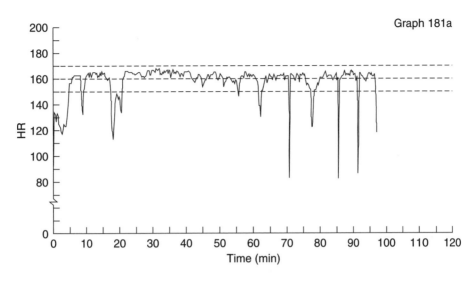

Graph 181a

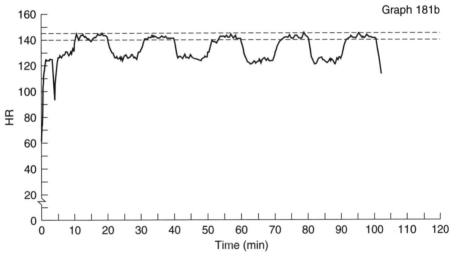

Graph 181b

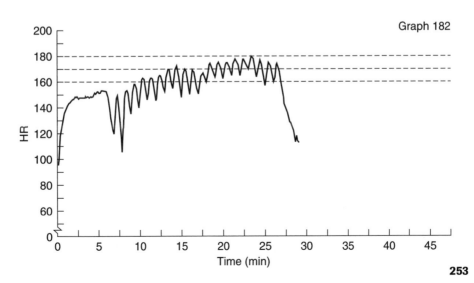

Graph 182

Test details

HRdefl: L4 = HR 165

Task: 20 × 10 seconds as intensive as possible, alternated by 50 seconds of recovery

Lactate after 10 times = 7.4 millimoles per liter

Lactate after 20 times = 9.8 millimoles per liter

For a workout with intensive repetitions, the intensity was correct. Lactate content reached a value between 6 and 12 millimoles per liter. Note that it took a long time before maximum HR (HRmax) was reached.

This kind of workout especially taxes lactate tolerance, as deduced from the high lactate concentrations reached. If the intention had been to train the CP system, this workout would have been too intensive. When training the CP system, such high lactate values must not be reached. These high lactate values could have been avoided by taking longer periods of recovery, so the phosphate system had more time to recharge. The first 6 minutes of the curve in graph 182 cover the warm-up.

Graph 183 shows an example workout of extensive repetitions during a cyclo-cross workout in the forest. The deflection point is L4 = HR 165. There are a number of time points with an intensity greater than HR 165. There are also long recovery periods. Lactate at the end of the workout was 10.2 millimoles per liter. So for an extensive workout, the intensity was too high. Graph 184 shows another example of intensive repetitions by a cyclist during a so-called overpass workout, in which maximum effort of 15 to 20 seconds was alternated with short recovery periods. The deflection point was L4 = HR 160. In this case, HRmax was reached gradually. So this was an intensive lactate tolerance workout in which high lactate values were reached.

The marathon runner's workout shown in graph 185 was a combination of an intensive endurance workout followed by extensive repetitions. The HRdefl was L4 = HR 144. There were three time units with an HR between 140 and 145 (intensive endurance) and then two units with an HR of about 150 (extensive tolerance). Between the units there was a long recovery pause. The first three units were the endurance 1 phase, and the last two units were the endurance 2 phase.

The next example is a team time trial by a 23-year-old pro cyclist in the Tour de France (graph 186). The first part was the warm-up. During the race, the cyclist rode 55 minutes above the level of L4 = HR 180.

Test details

L2 = HR 165, HRmax = 197

L3 = HR 175

L4 = HR 180

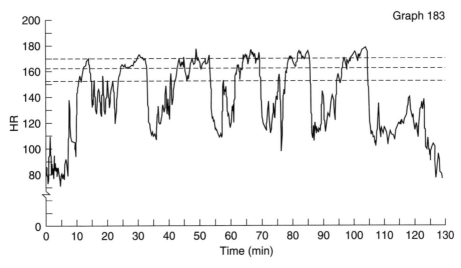

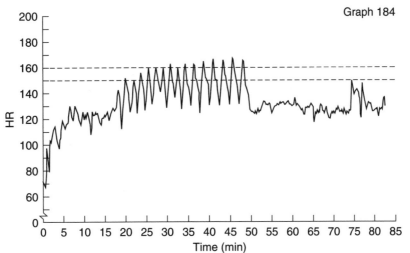

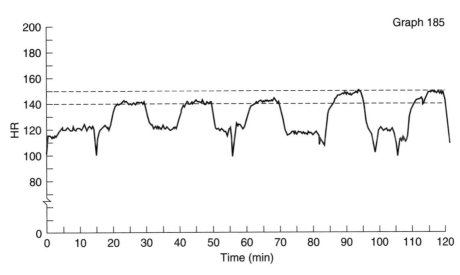

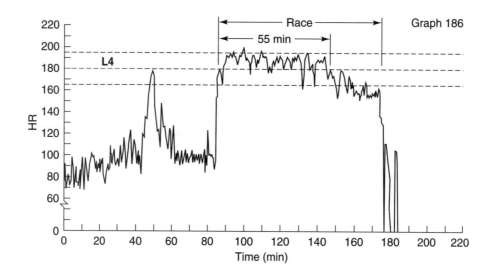

The cyclist's HRmax in the race was 197. After 55 minutes in the race he had reached maximum acidosis and was no longer capable of maintaining the speed of his teammates. Yet he kept performing to his maximum to finish within the time limit. If he had not succeeded he would have been out of the race. From a subjective point of view, he performed maximally, yet his HR and speed decreased. He rode above his HRdefl for too long. The curve quite clearly shows that well-trained persons may perform high in the anaerobic zone for quite some time.

The aerobic workout of a pro cyclist is shown in graph 187.

Test details

L2 = HR 150, HRmax = 175
L3 = HR 155
L4 = HR 160

The curve represents a workout intended to train endurance capacity. The workout was carried out in two different ways. First there were units with short recovery periods and then a constant pace without recovery periods.

This curve shows that the workout was correct for the aerobic system. During the working episodes, HR was between 150 and 160, so lactate was between L2 and L4.

A workout and time trial pattern of a 22-year-old pro cyclist are depicted in graphs 188 and 189. It was an intensive, and according to the rider, very heavy endurance workout.

The total workout lasted 7 hours. HR during the first 5.5 hours was between 110 and 120. So this workout was extensive, and especially fat oxidation was stimulated. The last part of the remaining 1.5 hours was an intensive lactate

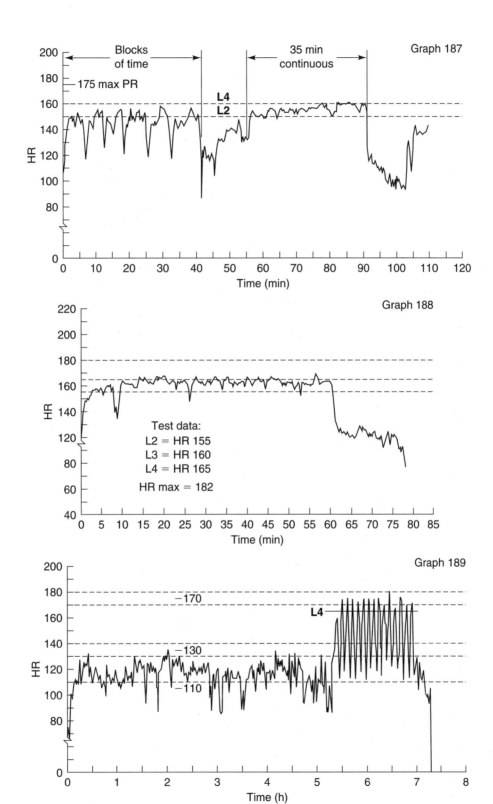

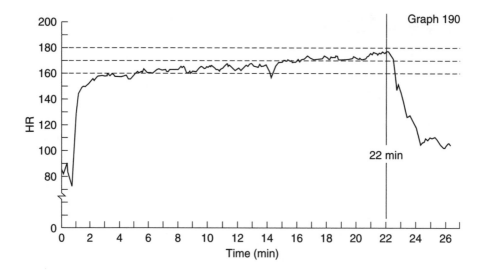

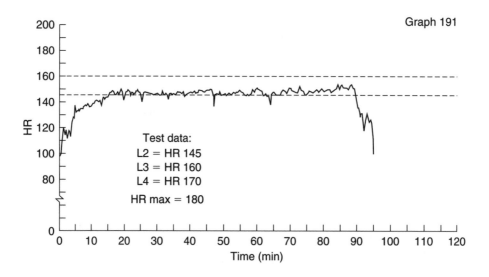

tolerance workout, in which a 1,200-meter climb was ridden 15 times at maximum speed.

In this 22-minute race, the HR gradually increased from 160 to nearly 180. The dip at the 14th minute (shown in graph 190) was a 180-degree turn in the race course. From this point onward there was a strong front wind and HR rapidly increased to more than 170. In the light of this rider's capabilities, the first 8 minutes were not optimal.

Graph 191 shows an extensive endurance workout by a triathlete. With these test data, the pattern is a good example of an extensive workout. The

HR constantly fluctuated between 145 and 150, just over L2 level. We can conclude that this was a correct extensive endurance workout.

Graphs 192 and 193 show two sprint workouts of a pro cyclist.

Test details

L2 = HR 150, HRmax = 175

L3 = HR 155

L4 = HR 160

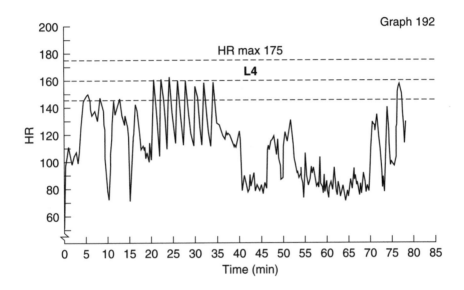

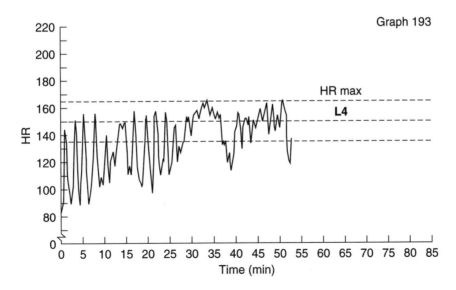

The task was to perform the sprint workout after warming up. The exercise phase was 10 to 20 seconds, and the recovery phase was 3 to 5 minutes. HR gradually increased to HRmax.

HR did not increase more than 160, possibly because there was insufficient recovery from the last workout. In addition, the recovery pauses were too short. In sprint workouts there should not be high lactate concentrations, so recovery pauses must be long. Sprint workouts only make sense when recovery is complete.

During sprint workouts, the HR gradually increases with every sprint, reaching HRmax by the end of the workout. In graphs 192 and 193, HRmax was not reached. Graph 194 shows an aerobic workout of a pro cyclist. The task was an aerobic workout in continuous units.

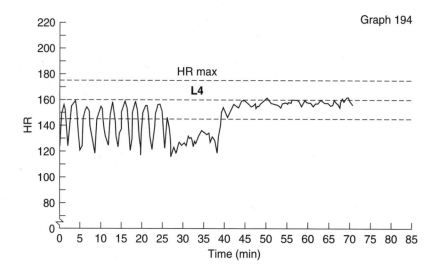

Graph 194

Test details

L2 = HR 150, HRmax = 175

L3 = HR 155

L4 = HR 160

The curve shows short exercise units, with a duration of 1 to 2 minutes, during which HR increased to 160. Recovery pauses were short, and HR decreased to 120. The curve also shows HR between 150 and 160 continuously (i.e., without breaks) during 30 minutes.

The first part of the workout was, in fact, an anaerobic workout, during which HR decreased to 120. In itself it was not a bad workout, but it did not meet the task.

During the unit workout, the exercise phases should be longer than 3 minutes—for example, up to 8 minutes. The continuous part was 20 to 60 minutes, which was sufficient. During that part HR was between 150 and 160, which was between L2 and L4.

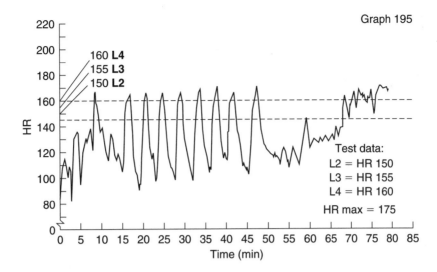

Graph 195

The curve in graph 195 represents a power workout of a pro cyclist The task was to remain seated on the saddle and ride uphill or in a front wind in top gear.

Test details

L2 = HR 150

L3 = HR 155

L4 = HR 160, HRmax = 175

Duration of the power phase was between 1 and 5 minutes. The number of repetitions was 4 to 10 times maximally. HR peaked over 160. The task was done well, and recovery was sufficient, during which HR rapidly decreased to 90. Graphs 196-214 show the HR patterns of athletes in various activities.

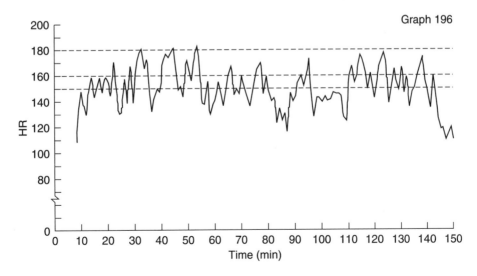

Graph 196

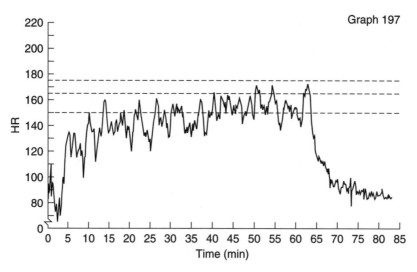

Graph 197

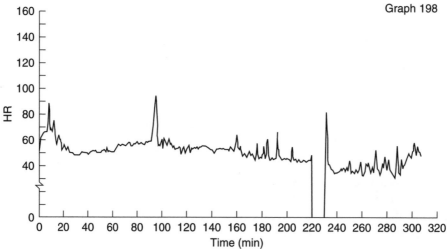

Graph 198

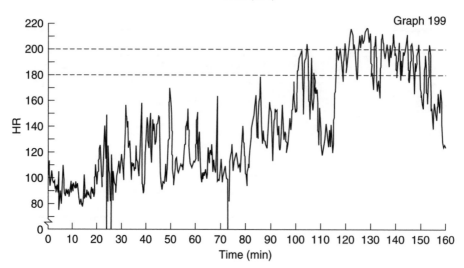

Graph 199

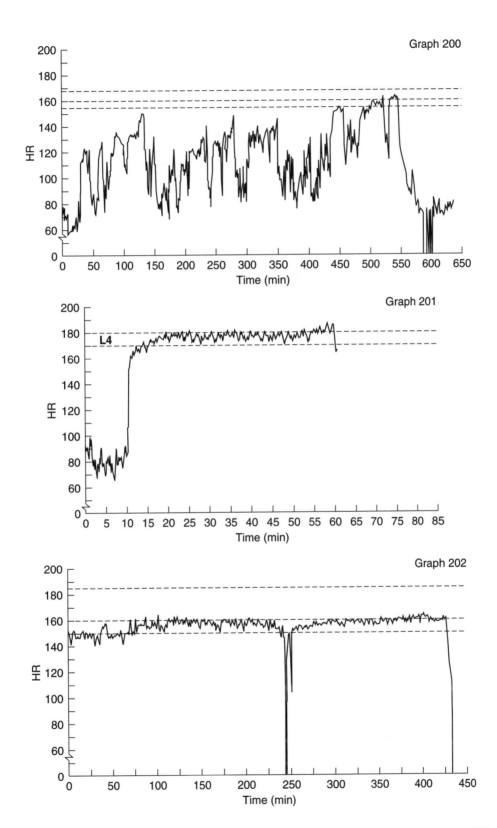

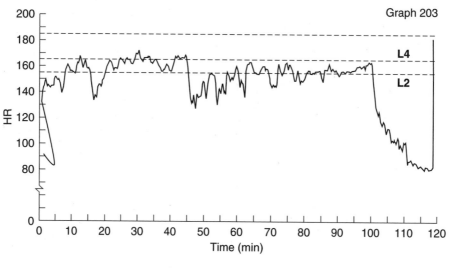

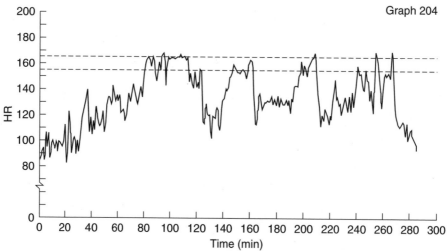

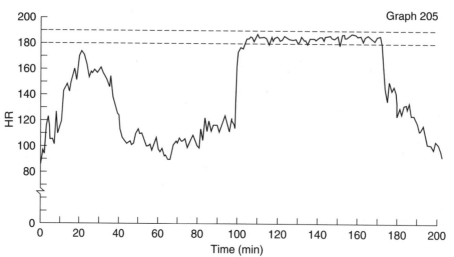

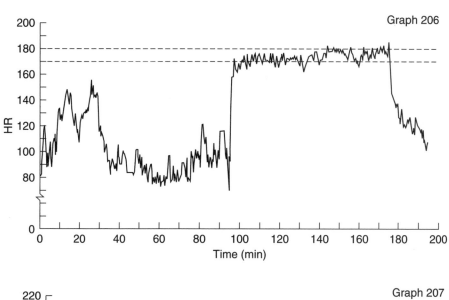

Graph 206

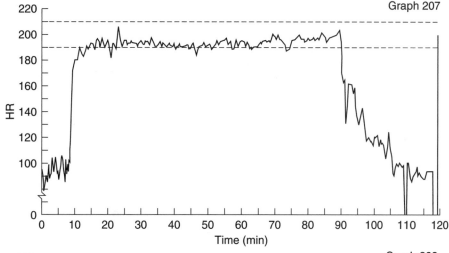

Graph 207

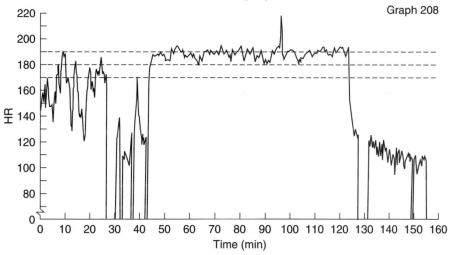

Graph 208

265

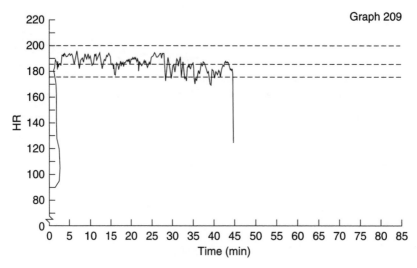

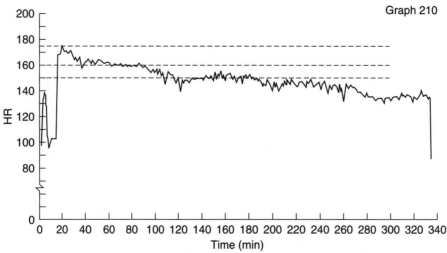

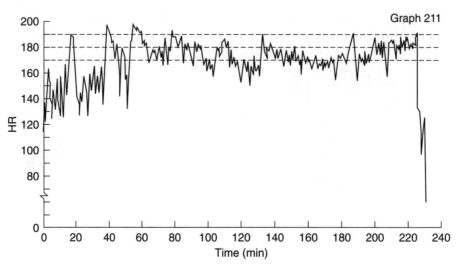

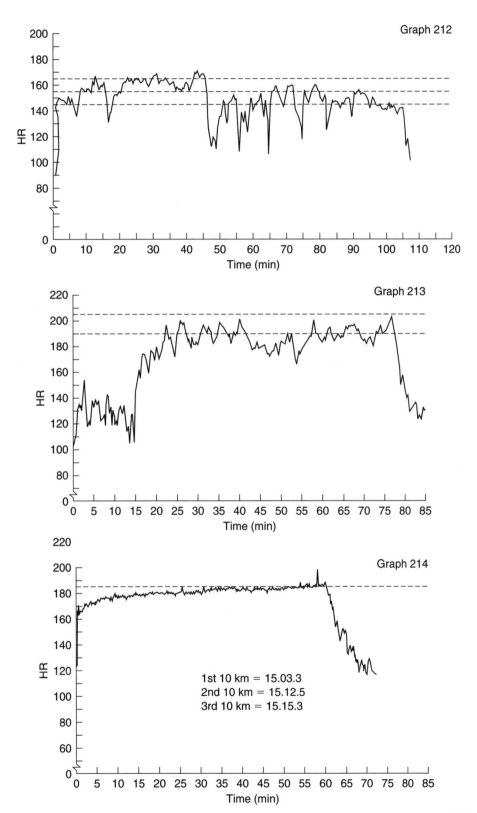

1st 10 km = 15.03.3
2nd 10 km = 15.12.5
3rd 10 km = 15.15.3

Sexual activity

There is a prejudice that sex before a race is disastrous to the male athlete in top condition. I have heard many discussions about the negative influence of a seminal discharge on performance capacity. There is also the belief that total sexual abstinence might evoke unknown powers; some athletes strongly believe that their victories are based on abstinence.

A prominent team leader of a cycling team once called me in the dead of night—panic in his voice—and urged me to approach a highly paid rider and advise total abstinence. The rider in question had jested on the massage table that he had had as many as three spontaneous seminal discharges during the night. It was not surprising that he rode poorly and had to let go of the pack at the first slope.

Intelligent top riders are so foolish as to abstain from having sex during the full early season (some 3 months). The most radical was the rider who slept with a very tight toe-clip strap around his penis to prevent it from discharging spontaneously during the night.

HR patterns made during sexual activity show that having sex equals a very light endurance workout for the trained athlete. However, it is unlikely that this information will dispel the prejudice that sex is disastrous before a race. If an athlete is convinced that sex before the race is bad, it will be difficult to change this belief. Like Lord Jeffrey once said, "Opinions based on prejudice are always defended with utmost ferocity."

Graph 215 shows the night and sex curve of a trained endurance athlete, and 216 shows the curve of an untrained person.

We can conclude that sex is equal to a light workout or recovery workout for a trained athlete. Also for an untrained person, sex is a submaximal effort.

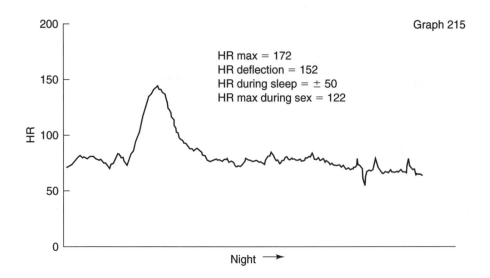

Graph 215

HR max = 172
HR deflection = 152
HR during sleep = ± 50
HR max during sex = 122

Night ⟶

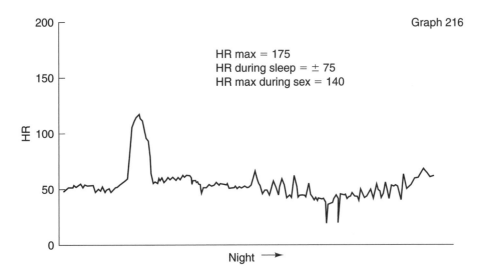

Graph 216

HR max = 175
HR during sleep = ± 75
HR max during sex = 140

200

150

HR 100

50

0

Night ⟶

HR patterns Through the Tour de France

The following graphs present an account of cyclist Eddy Bouwmans's experience in the 1995 Tour de France. Track his progress day by day and notice his HR compared with the topography.

HRdefl: 185 to 190

HR at rest: 45

HRmax: 200

Maximum power output: 500 to 545 watts

Weight: 69 to 72 kilograms

Fat percentage: 9.8% to 11.6%

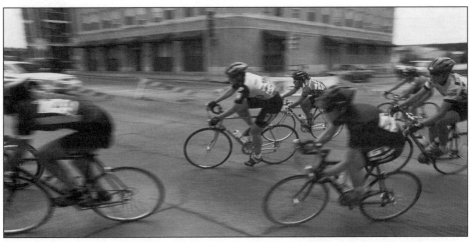

Cyclists can reach their maximum lactate potential by training their individual talents such as road-racing or cyclo-cross.

July 1

Prologue, 7.3 kilometers. Good night's sleep. HRrest = 45.

Onset: downhill, last 3 kilometers uphill.

20th pace: Ridden in dry weather.

The other competitors in rainy weather.

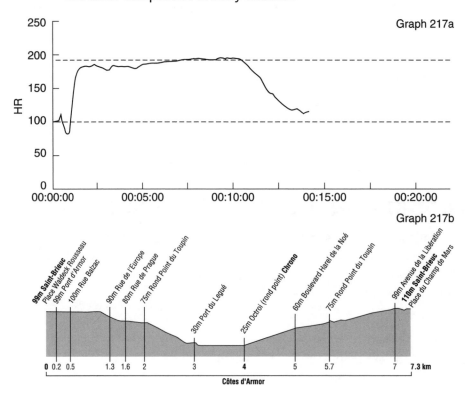

Graph 217a

Graph 217b

July 2

First stage, 233 kilometers. Good night's sleep. Rode fast in the last 50 kilometers only.

Average speed in the race, 40 kilometers per hour.

Uphill arrival, mass sprint.

Did not feel well; legs felt powerless.

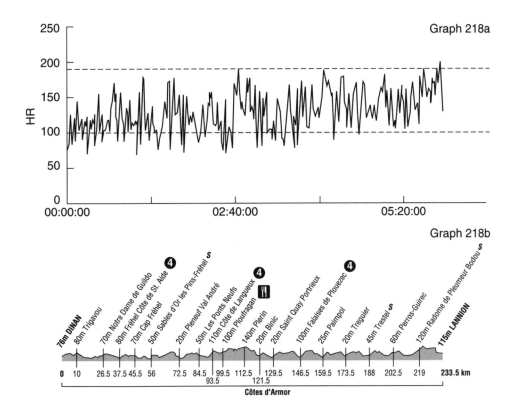

Graph 218a

Graph 218b

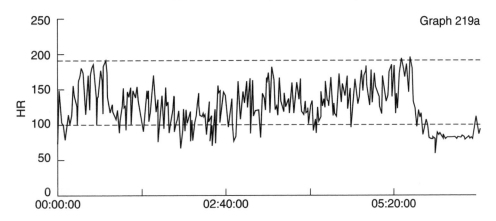

July 3

Second stage, 237 kilometers. Good night's sleep from 10 P.M. to 8 A.M. Rode well. Inattention made me miss decisive escape.

Rode fast. Average in the race 43.3 kilometers per hour.

Graph 219a

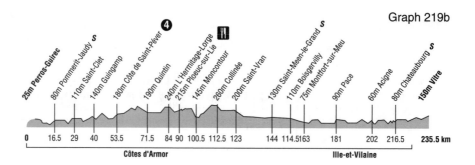

Graph 219b

**July
4**

Third stage, team time trial of 67 kilometers. Slept reasonably. HRrest = 51.
Rode reasonably well; experienced flat tire and time loss.
Could take the lead by the end.
Tenth place at 2 minutes 50 seconds from the winners.

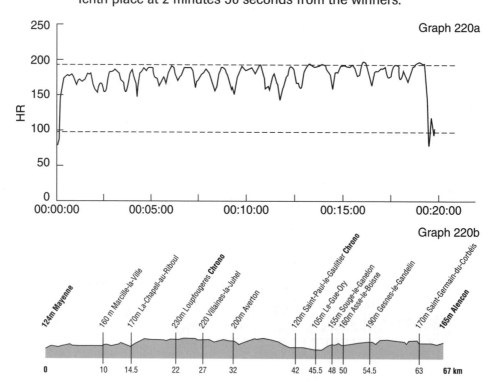

Graph 220a

Graph 220b

July 5
Fourth stage, 175 kilometers. Good night's sleep. HRrest = 49. Rather flat roads.

Rode rather well.

Somewhat sore legs due to the team time trial yesterday.

Mass sprint. Average speed in race = 44 kilometers per hour.

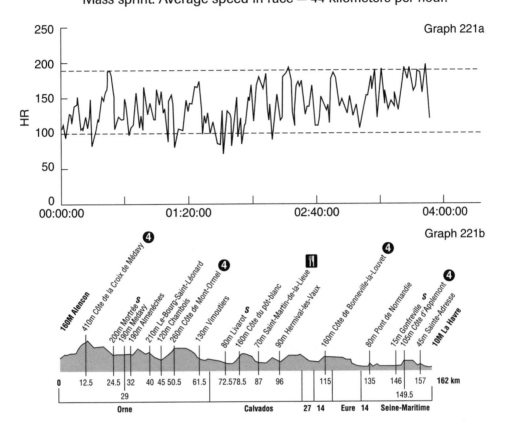

Graph 221a

Graph 221b

July 6
Fifth stage, 261 kilometers. Slept well. HRrest = 50.

Tailwind all day. Mass sprint.

Average speed = 45 kilometers per hour.

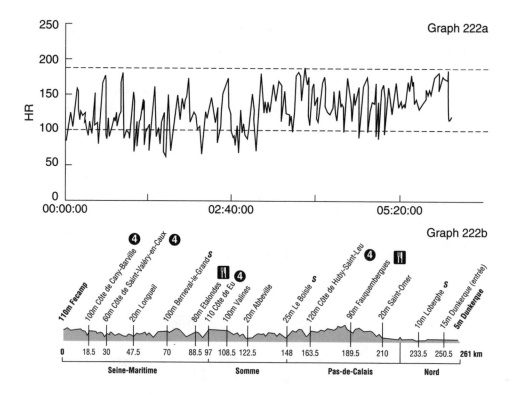

Graph 222a

Graph 222b

July 7	Sixth stage, 202 kilometers. Slept well. HRrest = 50. Flat roads. Rode well. Prepared sprints for Abdu. Average speed race: 44.7 kilometers per hour.

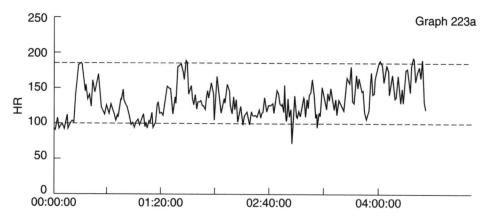

Graph 223a

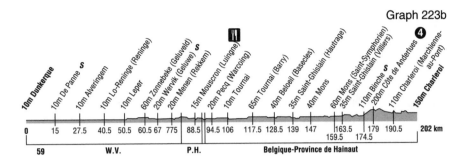

Graph 223b

July 8

Seventh stage, Belgian Ardennes. Slept well. HRrest = 50.
Not bad. The whole race was fast, especially uphill.
Occasional HR = 205.
Had to let go on the last slope.
Average speed race 42 kilometers per hour.

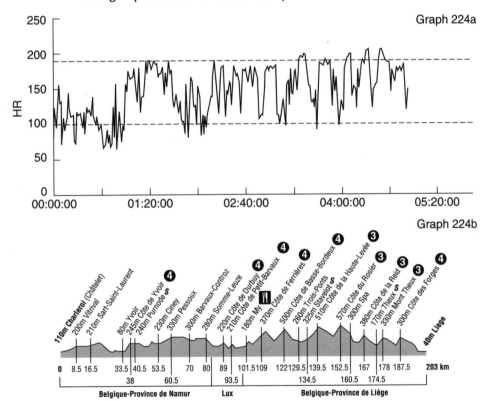

Graph 224a

Graph 224b

| July 9 | Eighth stage, time trial 54 km. Did not sleep well. HR = 51.
Went rather well. Time, 1 hour and 12 minutes at 7:57 from Indurain.
Painful buttock muscles. |
|---|---|

| July 10 | Traveling day. Slept reasonably well. HRrest = 50.
Bus ride to the hotel made me feel sick.
1.15 hours of light riding. |
|---|---|

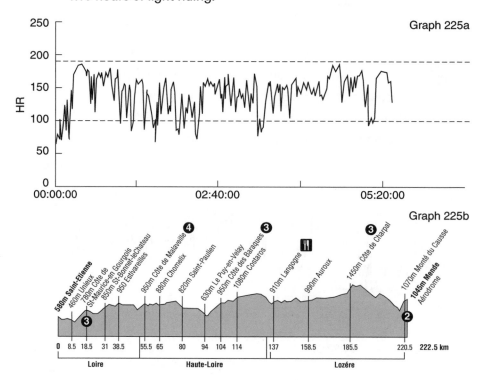

Graph 225a

Graph 225b

| July 11 | Ninth stage, 162 kilometers. Slept well. HRrest = 57.
Uphill arrival. Sore legs at the beginning.
Less sore later. After 40 kilometers I was in an escape group.
Had to let go on a slope later.
Arrived 20 minutes after the winner. |
|---|---|

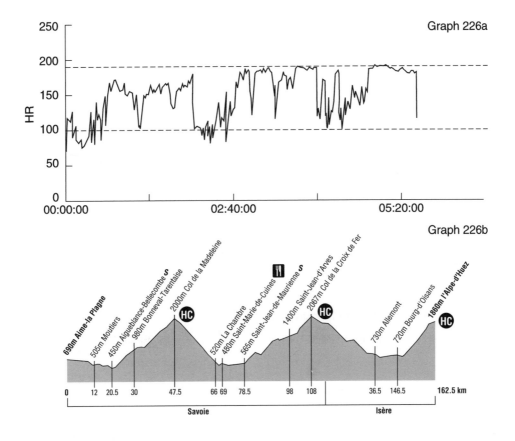

Graph 226a

Graph 226b

July 12 Tenth stage, 165 kilometers. Slept well. HRrest = 157.
Arrival at the Alpe d'Huez.
Went rather well, just like yesterday.
Collapsed some 9 kilometers before the arrival.
Too much effort in the beginning.

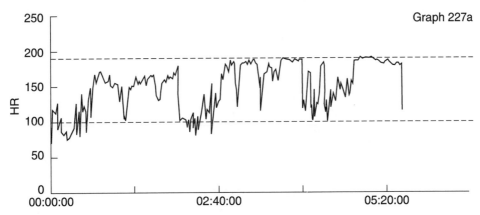

Graph 227a

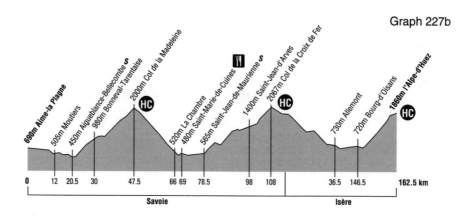

Graph 227b

July 13

Eleventh stage, 202 kilometers. Slept well. HRrest = 54.

In the beginning I did not feel well.

Later on it was better.

Could take the lead in favor of Abdu.

Average racing speed race = 41.5 kilometers per hour.

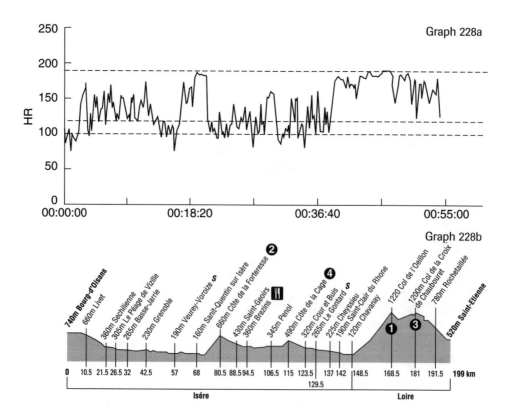

Graph 228a

Graph 228b

July 14

Twelfth stage, 232 kilometers. Slept well. HRrest = 52.
Troublesome and heavy day.
By the end we had to take the lead; I don't quite understand why.
Jalabert was far ahead and Abdu could not win anyway.
The final was too difficult.

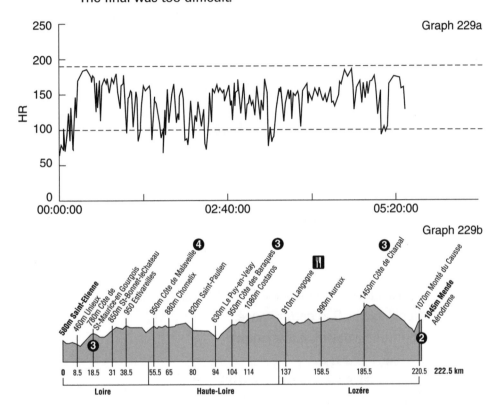

Graph 229a

Graph 229b

July 15

Thirteenth stage, 245 kilometers. Slept well. HRrest = 56.
In the beginning, very high speed (downhill).
Did not feel well. Could not join the leading group of 30.
Later on in the race things went better.

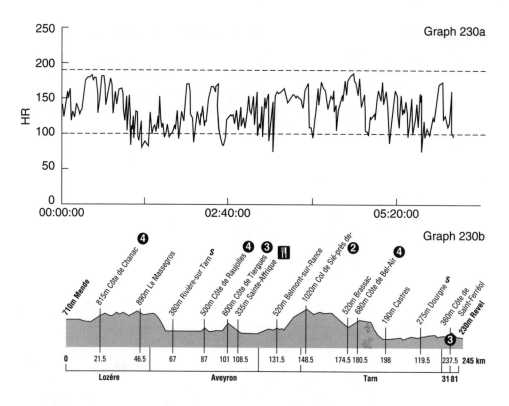

July 16
Fourteenth stage, 164 kilometers. Did not sleep well.
Uphill arrival. Bad performance.
Fortunately, day of rest tomorrow.

July 17
Day of rest. Slept reasonably. HRrest = 50.
Rested. Photo session for the press.
Some light riding.

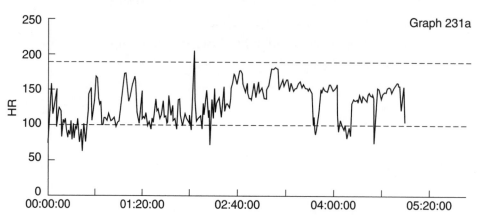

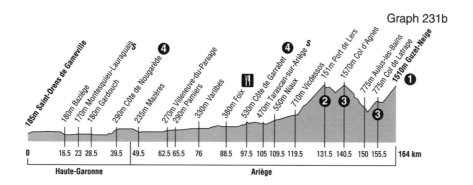

Graph 231b

July 18

Fifteenth stage, 206 kilometers. Slept well. HRrest = 50.

The star stage with uphill arrival.

Bad legs in the first two mountain passes.

Had to let go on the Tourmalet, 10 kilometers before summit.

On the last slope (very steep), no more maximum effort.

After arrival, I heard that Fabio Casartelli died in hospital after a fall.

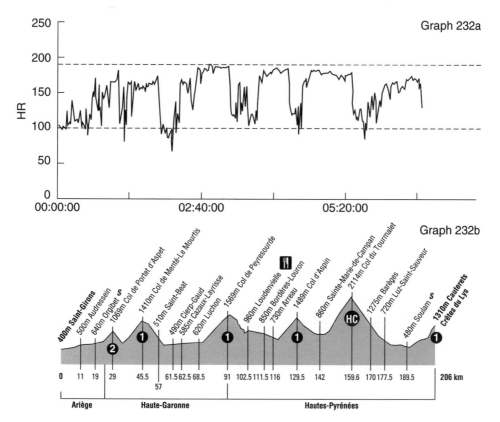

Graph 232a

Graph 232b

July 19

Sixteenth stage, 237 kilometers. Slept reasonably. HRrest = 52.

Fabio's death burdens me.

I did start but did not ride fast in honor of Fabio.

The route was fairly troublesome, although none of us really rode.

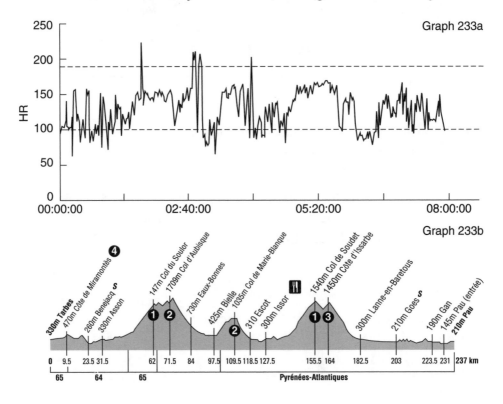

Graph 233a

Graph 233b

July 20

Seventeenth stage, 246 kilometers. Slept reasonably. HRrest = 52.

Did not feel well.

No HR recording.

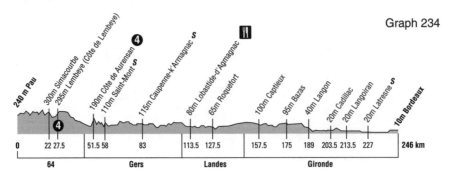

Graph 234

July 21

Eighteenth stage, 169 kilometers. Slept well. HRrest = 55.

Things went bad all day.

Could stay in the pack only with difficulty.

Diarrhea in the evening.

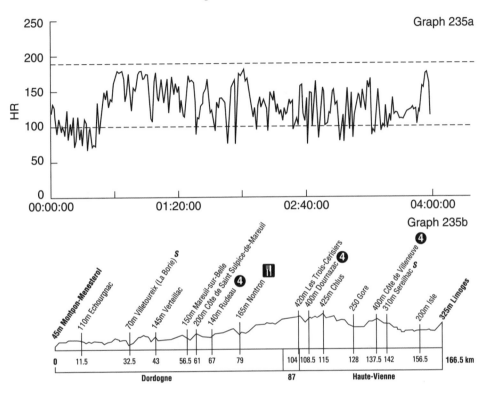

Graph 235a

Graph 235b

July 22

Ninteenth stage, 47-kilometer individual time trial. Bad sleep.

Things went reasonably well, in spite of diarrhea.

My time: 01:05:46

Indurain: 57 minutes

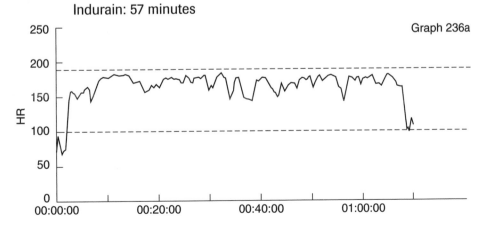

Graph 236a

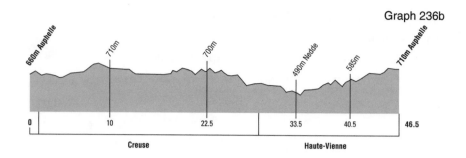

Graph 236b

| July 23 | Twentieth stage, 115 kilometers. Slept reasonably. Still have diarrhea. Did not ride well. |

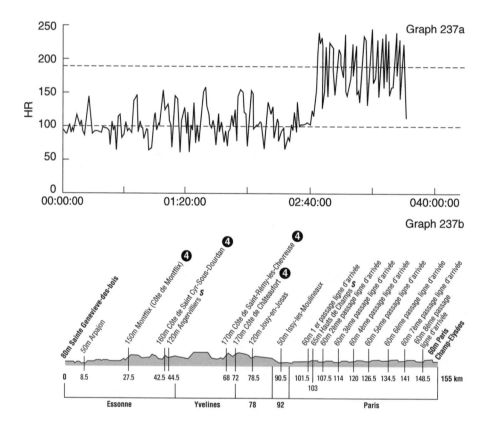

Graph 237a

Graph 237b

epilogue

Training analyses as well as the research literature show that training is often done at the wrong intensities. Athletes often do not understand or feel their training tasks. The methods described here provide a useful tool for teaching the athlete to listen to the signals of his or her body. With practice, one can learn the feeling of the right intensity. Athletes who use this tool are capable of performing at an accuracy of 0.5 millimoles per liter. So once you know the feeling of running or riding at a lactate concentration of 4 millimoles per liter, you are able to set the right intensity next time. The workload intensity may be divided subjectively on a scale from 1 to 5.

Workload intensity

> 1 = very light
>
> 2 = light
>
> 3 = medium
>
> 4 = heavy
>
> 5 = very heavy

It has been shown repeatedly that the assessment of workload intensity is very constant in the same person. Those with more training experience are better able to assess the intensity subjectively, once they have learned to do so.

The workload intensity of 4 millimoles of lactate per liter is felt as medium. When condition improves, the athlete's actual performance will be better at that lactate level, but the intensity still will be felt as medium. Once the athlete has learned to assess intensities correctly, this may be a perfect tool for optimizing training.

The optimal training load of 2 to 4 millimoles of lactate per liter applies not only to top athletes but to anyone engaged in sports. Mostly it is the medium-level and recreational athletes also who often use the wrong training methods, so that they reach complete exhaustion. Such an activity does not bring about the desired adaptations of the body that might lead to better performance.

In a study of 50 recreational runners, selected at random without previous information, lactate values of 6 to 12 millimoles per liter were found, the average being 8.5 millimoles per liter. Starting from an anaerobic threshold of 4 millimoles per liter, they all had 100% too much lactate. The same result was obtained in recreational swimmers. To make maximum profit of the body's adaptation capability, it is vitally important to maintain the recommended lactate thresholds. For the recreational runner this will mean running without becoming short of breath. Because recreational athletes may not have the opportunity to have their lactate levels checked, they must rely on heart rate measurement.

The training load for endurance sports should lead to heart rates of roughly 130 to 160 beats per minute in normal healthy men and women under 50. Those over 50 should use the following rule: Train at a heart rate of 180 minus your age in years. The exercise should last for 30 to 40 minutes for running, cycling, swimming, and so forth. Following this program three to four times a week, the individual trains in a healthy and responsible way.

Many sports are suitable for a fitness program. Choosing one that is enjoyable makes the task easier. Following are some of the best sports to keep fit:

Jogging	Tennis
Cycling	Basketball
Cross-country skiing	Football
Long-distance walking	Handball
Swimming	Rowing

A correct training progression takes the various energy-supplying systems as a starting point. These systems are the phosphate system and the lactate system, which supply anaerobic energy, and the glucose and fat oxidation system, which supplies aerobic energy.

Which system supplies the energy depends on the intensity and duration of exercise. Roughly speaking, short and fierce power bursts are supplied with anaerobic energy, and long-lasting exercise of intermediate intensity is supplied with aerobic energy. Each system is trained in a specific manner. Besides the training program that is targeted at a certain energy system, there should be enough time for sufficient recovery after the workouts.

The training program should be aimed first at improving aerobic endurance. The correct intensity for improving aerobic endurance is in the range of the aerobic-anaerobic transition zone, in the area between 2 and 4 millimoles of lactate per liter. Later, when aerobic endurance is trained sufficiently, the phosphate system and the lactate system can be stressed specifically.

The various types of workout should be worked into a total training program coherently and in the right doses. If one single type of workout gets too much attention, total performance capacity will suffer. Many athletes have problems with the right composition of the training program, making major mistakes in both in quality and quantity. The reason for these mistakes is that the athletes simply do not know at what intensity they are training. By setting the training tasks more precisely, according to the methods discussed in this book, it is possible to teach athletes the feeling of training at a certain intensity.

This feeling can be learned to an accuracy of 0.5 millimoles per liter, so then the athlete knows exactly how it feels to train at a lactate content of 2, 4, 6, or 10 millimoles per liter. Athletes often misjudge intensities, and the too-intensive workouts, done too often, in which high lactate concentrations are reached, negatively affect performance capacity. These programs still occur too often.

The athlete who wants to reach maximum performance tends to train too intensely and is only satisfied when the intensity of workouts approaches that of races. This feeling of "going for it" is caused by high lactate concentrations, which can reach values between 10 and 20 millimoles per liter. When the training program is this intense, the athlete will not reach the desired level of performance despite all of his or her efforts. The athlete then tends to increase training activities in an effort to reach that performance level, which further decreases performance and can lead to overtraining.

Acidosis, which is caused by high muscle lactate values, damages the aerobic enzymes system. This system may be seen as a factory where aerobic energy supply is generated. Thus, acidosis deteriorates aerobic capacity. After a heavy workout with high lactate concentrations, the body needs some time to repair the damaged aerobic enzymes system. Therefore, a light recovery workout is always advisable the day after a heavy workout.

Various sports require fine-tuned coordination together with a large aerobic capacity. Coordination should be trained separately. In most sports, coordination training is called technique training or technical skills training. Training coordination is seriously disturbed at lactate values higher than 8 millimoles per liter, and intricate technical skills cannot be performed. The higher the lactate content, the more problems with complicated technical skills. This is true in football, tennis, skating, hockey, wrestling, basketball, rowing, cyclo-cross, and many other sports.

We have seen that intensive workouts cause high lactate concentrations, which in turn decrease aerobic capacity and disturb coordination. In addition, the chance of injuries is higher during intensive workouts, because acidosis in the muscles causes microscopic damage to the muscle tissue. These minor damages, if not allowed sufficient recovery, can lead to more serious injuries.

Group workouts in various sports are often ineffective, because training tasks for the complete group might have a different effect on individual members. One athlete might train his anaerobic system, whereas another works on her aerobic capacity. A third one might even do a recovery workout. The trainer/coach should be aware of these limitations of group workouts. It is the task of the trainer/coach to adapt the workouts to benefit every individual member.

A final word: Heart rate measurement with or without lactate determination is an excellent method of assessing training intensities. This method is inexpensive and available to recreational as well as elite athletes.

glossary

acidosis—Lactate accumulation in the muscle cells.

ADP—Adenosine diphosphate.

aerobic-anaerobic transition zone—Energy supply within this range is both aerobic and anaerobic. The production and neutralization of lactate are in equilibrium. The area is between 2 and 4 millimoles per liter.

aerobic energy supply—Energy supply with sufficient oxygen: no lactate accumulation.

aerobic threshold—Any exercise up to this level is fully aerobic. Lactate concentration at the aerobic threshold is about 2 millimoles per liter.

alactic anaerobic endurance—During exercise the body is capable of maximum work for 10 to 20 seconds without oxygen. The energy comes from high-energy phosphates (ATP and CP). There is no lactate production.

anaerobic endurance—The capacity of muscles to keep performing without sufficient oxygen.

anaerobic energy supply—Energy supply with insufficient oxygen, which results in a lactate accumulation.

anaerobic lactic endurance—During intensive exercise, with insufficient oxygen, lactate production will start after 10 to 20 seconds. Within this workload, the highest values are reached after 60 to 180 seconds.

anaerobic threshold—Exercise above this level brings about a strong acidosis. The lactate concentration at the anaerobic threshold is about 4 millimoles per liter in most athletes, although some have higher values.

Åstrand bicycle ergometer test—In an Åstrand test, condition is determined by counting HR during one submaximal effort. It is a fast and easy method of determining $\dot{V}O_2$max.

ATP—Adenosine triphosphate, a high-energy compound.

bpm—Beats per minute.

Calorie (or kilocalorie) —The amount of heat required to warm up 1 gram of water by 1 degree Celsius. One kilocalorie = 4.2 kilojoules, so the conversion factor is 4.2.

Conconi test—A noninvasive test (i.e., without blood sampling) to determine the deflection pulse or deflection pace. The test is based on the relationship between HR and pace.

condition—The physical and psychological state of an athlete. Aspects of condition are endurance capacity, strength, speed, coordination, flexibility, techniques, and tactics. The psychological aspect also plays a role.

condition determination—Determining an athlete's condition is based on the linear relation between HR and intensity of exercise. In an Åstrand test, condition is determined on the basis of HR during one submaximal effort. It is a fast and simple method that enables $\dot{V}O_2$max determination. The $\dot{V}O_2$max is expressed in liters per minute. The higher the $\dot{V}O_2$max, the better the condition.

CP—Creatine phosphate (or phosphocreatine), a high-energy phosphate present in muscle cells. During maximum effort, the high-energy phosphates (ATP and CP) are depleted after 10 to 20 seconds.

Dp—deflection pulse; HR at the HRdefl. Training may cause the Dp to shift to a higher level, which means that you can perform at a higher HR without lactate accumulation. To do so you should have regular workouts around the Dp, which are fairly strenuous workouts. Because this Dp may shift, it should be determined periodically.

ergometer—Apparatus on which exercise tests are done (e.g., bicycle ergometer, running belt, etc.)

extensive/intensive—Two terms often used in a comparative sense. Extensive means costing little energy per time unit, often of longer duration or more repetitions. Intensive means costing much energy per time unit, often of shorter duration or fewer repetitions.

fatigue—Signals of fatigue include waking up and still being tired, heightened morning pulse, bad sleep, irritability, no eagerness for workouts, and "heavy" legs. HR does not rise or hardly rises during exercise. Blood sampling shows heightened values. No single signal indicates fatigue. It is always better to skip a heavy workout when fatigued.

glucose—A sugar; one of the most important carbohydrates.

glycogen—The form in which glucose is stored in the body.

HR—Heart rate.

HRdefl—the deflection point, the point at which the linear relation between HR and intensity of exercise is lost; also known as the anaerobic threshold.

HRmax—Maximum HR; the formula of the HRmax (220 minus age in years) often does not apply. The same person might have different HRmax values for different sports. The HRmax decreases as age increases. HRmax may decrease by four to six beats after a period of intensive training. Always determine HRmax several times. The highest value is the real HRmax.

HR monitor—Device that includes a chest belt from which a signal is emitted. This chest belt registers the electric pulses of the heart and sends them to a receiver, which is worn as a wristwatch or attached to the bars of a bike. The actual HR can be seen on the receiver at any moment. There are advanced HR monitors with various functions: for example, allowing the athlete to pre-set limits, or beeping when HR is too high or too low. A data memory bank enables the user to plot HR curves of workouts or races for later analysis. It is especially for that function that the HR monitor has become an essential instrument in modern sports coaching.

HR recovery after exercise—When the athlete is in good condition, the HR will decrease by 30 to 40 beats in the first minute after stopping the exercise (e.g., intervals). This decrease in HR is largest in the first minute; later it will be slower.

HR reserve—The difference between HRmax and HRrest.

HRrest—HR at rest; this is preferably established in the morning, before getting up (which is why it is also called morning pulse). Count your heartbeat for 30 seconds and multiply by two. That is your HRrest.

IAT—Individual anaerobic threshold.

intensive/extensive—See extensive/intensive.

Karvonen—A Finnish sports physiologist who developed the method of the HR reserve. This method uses certain percentages of this reserve.

L—Lactate or lactic acid; a by-product of glucose oxidation with insufficient oxygen supply (anaerobic energy supply).

MLSS—Maximal lactate steady state; the highest intensity at which no lactate will accumulate.

phosphate battery—The total amount of high-energy phosphates ATP and CP.

RPM—Revolutions per minute.

threshold pace—Pace at the HRdefl. It is also called V4 pace and corresponds with the Dp.

tolerance workouts—High-intensity workouts in the lactate formation zone.

training intensities—This book has adopted the new international designations of the various intensity zones. Roughly speaking there are three zones: the aerobic zone, the endurance zone, and the anaerobic zone. In the aerobic zone, energy supply comes from purely aerobic processes. The endurance zone is just under and just over the anaerobic threshold, so energy supply is partially aerobic and partially anaerobic. The anaerobic zone is based on energy supply without sufficient oxygen intake, which may lead to lactate accumulation. If the exercise is one power burst of about 10 seconds, the high-energy phosphates will be called on.

The three zones are subdivided in two areas:

A1 aerobic 1, the intensity is very low, about 70% to 80% of the anaerobic threshold.

A2 aerobic 2, the intensity is somewhat higher, 80% to 90% of the anaerobic threshold.

E1 endurance 1, in the transition zone, 90% to 100% of the anaerobic threshold.

E2 endurance 2, high-intensity endurance, 100% to 110% of the anaerobic threshold.

An1 anaerobic 1, based on anaerobic glycolysis, maximum energy supply 2 to 3 minutes.

An2 anaerobic 2, pure power bursts like sprints and weight lifting. No lactate formation.

V4—The pace or speed at a lactate content of 4 millimoles per liter. On the basis of the V4, exact training advice can be given.

$\dot{V}O_2$max—Maximum oxygen uptake in liters per minute.

bibliography

Abraham, P., G. Leftheriotis, Y. Bourre, J. M. Chevalier, and J. L. Saumet. 1993. Echography of external iliac artery endofibrosis in cyclists. *American Journal of Sports Medicine* 2:861-863.

Afzien: de ontwikkeling van het werelduurrecord. 1981. *Verenigingsorgaan van de Medische Wielerkring Nederland (MWN)* 11:13.

Althof, Q., and A. van Geel. 1993. *Goede voeding, de beste taktische zet*. Kruiswerk West-Brabant: Thuiszorg Midden-Brabant.

American College of Sports Medicine. 1994. *Resource manual for guidelines for exercise testing and prescription*. Philadelphia: Lea & Febiger.

Anderson, O. 1996. Eten en drinken. *Runner's World* April, 18-19.

Arts in beweging. Sportmedisch informatieblad van de Ned. Ver. Van trimmende artsen. 1992. *Vrouw en Sport* 8(18).

Åstrand, P. O. *Work tests with the bicycle ergometer*. Sweden: Monark-Crescent AB.

Åstrand, P. O., and K. Rodahl. 1986. *Textbook of work physiology*. New York: McGraw-Hill.

Berge Henegouwen, D. P. van. 1992. Claudicatio intermittans bij jeugdige patienten (ingezonden brief). *Nederlands Tijdschrift voor Geneeskunde* 136(24):1176.

Berglund, B. 1992. High-altitude training. *Sports Medicine* 14(5):289-303.

Binkhorst, R. 1981. Anaërobe drempel. *Geneeskunde en Sport* 3:78-79.

Bosch, J. van den. 1989. De test van Conconi in de praktijk. *Atletiekwereld*, 4, March 28, 23-26.

Boverman, B. 1991. *Richting Sportgericht* 45:6. "Marathontraining met Gelindo Bordin."

Brick, M. 1984. *Precision multisport*. Finland: Uitgeverij Polar Electro Oy.

Brok, A. G. M. T. 1995. Doping, de stand van zaken. *Geneeskunde en Sport* 28(6):162-168.

Brok, A. G. M. F. 1995. Inspanning, infectie en immuniteit. *Geneeskunde en Sport* 28(6):178-181.

Brouns, F. 1993. *Nutritional needs of athletes*. Chichester, UK: Wiley.

Bush, T. L., L. D. Cowan, E. Barrett-Connor, M. H. Crique, J. M. Karon, R. B. Wallace, H. A. Tyroler, and B. M. Rifkind. 1983. Estrogen use and all-cause mortality. *Journal of the American Medical Association* 249:903-906.

Carella, M., D'Ambrosio, L., et. al. 1997. Mutation analysis of the HCAH gene in Italian hemochromatosis patients. *Am. J. Hum. Gen.* 60:828-832.

Chevalier, J. M. 1989. L'endofibrose iliaque externe du cycliste de competition. In Technopathies du cyclisme, edited by J. P. de Mondenard. Frankrijk: Uitgave van Ciba-Geigy.

Chevalier, J. M., Enon, J. Walder, X. Barrel, J. Pillet, A. Megret, P. L'Hoste, J. P. Saint-Andre, and M. Davinroy. 1986. Endofibrosis of the external iliac artery in bicycle racers: An unrecognized pathological state. *Annals of Vascular Surgery* 1:297-303.

Chevalier, J. M., P. L'Hoste, E. Bouvat, A. Megret, J. P. Saint Andre, and P. Ruault. 1991. L' endofibrose arterielle du sportif de haut niveau: Formes inhabituelles. *Journal of Traumatology in Sport* 8:176-181.

Claes, J. 1984. Een evaluatie van BE bepalingen. *Sportmedische Tijdingen* 2045-2061.

Clarke, D. V. 1986. Sex differences in strength and fatigability. *Research Quarterly in Exercise and Sport* 57:144-149.

Clarys, J. P., et al. 1985. Wielrennen. Lochem-Gent: Uitgeverij De Tijdstroom.

Conconi, F., M. Ferrari, P. Ziglio, P. Droghetti, and L. Codeca. 1982. Determination of the anaerobic threshold by a noninvasive field test in runners. *Journal of Applied Physiology* 52:869-873.

Couwenhoven, R. 1994. Column. *Wielerrevue* 23/24.

Coyle, E. F. 1994. Fluid and carbohydrate replacement during exercise; How much and why? *Sports Science Exchange* 7(3).

Coyle, E. F. 1995. Integration of the physiological factors determining endurance performance ability. *Exercise and Sport Sciences Reviews* 23:25-63.

Edwards, S. 1994. Trainen met een hartslagmeter. *Antennestraat* 46:1322.

Eichner, E. R. 1984. The exercise hypothesis: An updated analysis. In *Year Book of Sports Medicine*, edited by L. J. Krakauer, J. L. Anderson, and R. J. Shepard. Chicago: Year Book Medical.

Eichner, E. R. 1988. A profile of the mature athlete. *Advances in Sports Medicine and Fitness* 1:1-22.

Ekblom, B. 1986. Applied physiology of soccer. *American Journal of Sports Medicine* 3:50-60.

Erp-Baart, A. M. J. van. 1985. *Inspanning en voeding*. Alphen aan de Rijn/Brussels, Belgium: Uitgeverij Samson/Staflieu.

Fagard, R. 1995. De betekenis van linker-ventrikelhypertrofie voor de atleet. Paper presented at the Symposium Het Sporthart, de grijze zone in de cardiologie van het Cardiovasculair Onderwijs Instituut, 1 December, Zeist, The Netherlands.

Faraggiana, D. 1991. Lecture presented at the 16th congress of the European Athletics Coaches Association, 17-21 January, Vierumaki, Finland.

Fox, E., and D. Matthews. 1991. Fysiologie van lichamelijke inspanning en sport. Lochem: De Tijdstroom.

Fox, E. L., and D. K. Matthews. *The Physiological Basis of Physical Education and Athletics.*

Fry, R. W., A. R. Morton, and D. Keast. 1991. Overtraining in athletes. *Sports Medicine* 12:32-65.

Geijsel, J. 1986. Triatlontotaal. Utrecht, The Netherlands: Uitgeverij Kosmos.

Geijsel, J. 1990. Het trappen op volle toeren. *Support Personal Magazine* 3: (Available from Uitgave van Support, Antennestraat 46, 1322 AS Almere, The Netherlands)

Geijsel, J. 1994. Lactaatdynamica. *Geneeskunde en Sport* 27(5):165-169.

Hartgens, F., and P. G. J. M. Janssen. 1994. Arteria iliaca externa bij wielrenners. *Geneeskunde en Sport* 27(6):185-188.

Havenith, G. 1996. Atlanta 1996: Praktische aanwijzingen voor inspanning in de hitte. *Geneeskunde en Sport* 29(1):16-21.

Heck, H. 1985. Justification of the 4-mmol/lactate threshold. *International Journal of Sports Medicine* 6:117-130.

Heck, H., G. Hess, and A. Mader. 1985. Vergleichende Untersuchung zu verschiedenen Lactat-Schwellenkonzepten. *Deutsche Zeitschrift für Sportmedizin* 36:19-25.

Heide, L. de, and B. P. Hazenberg. 1994. Mononucleosis infectiosa, anders dan meestal. *Nederlands Tijdschrift van Geneeskunde* 131:2281-2283.

Hendriks, E. R. H. A., et al. 1992. *Leerboek Sportgeneeskunde*. Bohn, Staflieu, Van Loghum, Houten

Hoest, P. van der. 1999. De medische knipselkrant. 4 January. Titel: Een ijzersterke ziekte.

Hofmann, P., and G. Gaisl. 1988. Der Coconi-Test und seine praktische Anwendung. *Condition* 19(7):18-19.

Hollmann, W. 1986. Historical remarks on the development of the aerobic-anaerobic threshold. *International Journal of Sports Medicine* 6:109-116.

Hollmann, W. 1980. *Sportmedizin-, Arbeits- und Trainungsgrundlagen.* Stuttgart/New-York: F. K. Schattauer Verlag.

Hollmann, W., et al 1986. Die aerobe Leistungsfähigkeit—Aspekte von Gesundheit und Sport. *Spektrum der Wissenschaft*: 48-58.

Hoogsteen, J., and M. Huige. 1994. Het sporthart. *Janssen Medisch-Wetenschappelijk Nieuws* May 1994. (Available from Uitgave van Janssen Pharm., Postbus 90240, 5000 LT Tilburg, The Netherlands)

Hottenrott, K. 1993. *Trainingssteuerung im Ausdauersport.* Ahrensburg bei Hamburg, Germany: Verlag Ingrid Czwalina.

Houtmann, I., and H. Schlatmann. 1988. Fysiologie voor de Sportpraktijk. Lochem: Uitgeverij de Tijdstroom.

Hultman, E., J. Bergstrom, and N. M. Anderson. 1967. Breakdown and resynthesis of phosphorylcreatine and adenosinetriphosphate in connection with muscular work in man. *Scandinavian Journal of Clinical and Laboratory Investigation* 19:56-66.

Israel, S., and J. Weber. 1972. *Probleme der langzeit Ausdauer im Sport.* Leipzig, Germany: Johann Ambrosius Barth.

Jablonski, D., H. Liesen, I. Kraus, and H. Modder. 1985. Intesitätssteuerung und Leistungsbeurteilung beim Jogging. *Fortschritte der Medizin* 103(4):47-50.

Janssen, P. 1993. *Basisboek Training,* 5th ed. Utrecht, The Netherlands: Uitgeverij Kosmos Utrecht.

Jeukendrup, A., W. H. M. Saris, and F. Brouns. 1994. Substraatgebruik tijdens inspanning: De rol van vetten. *Geneeskunde en sport* 27(40):116-124.

Kanter, M. 1995. Free radicals and exercise: Effects of nutritional antioxidant supplementation. *Exercise and Sport Sciences Reviews* 23:349-398.

Kapsenberg, J. 1988. Moe van de virussen. *Nederlands Tijdschrift van geneeskunde* 132:997-999.

Karvonen, J. *Medicine in sports training and coaching.* Medicine and Sport Science, Vol. 35. Basel, Switzerland: Karger.

Kemper, H. C. G. 1990. *Fysiologie achtergronden van lichamelijke opvoeding en sport. Deel 1 en 2.* Uitgeverij De Vrieseborch, Haarlem. Deel 1: Basiskennis; deel 2: Toegepaste kennis.

Klooster, L. van 1996. De geheimen van Ferrari. *Fiets* 1:22-24.

Kloosterboer, T., et al. 1993 *Elementaire trainingsleer en trainingsmethoden.* Haarlem, The Netherlands: De Vrieseborch.

Krauss, R.M. 1989. Exercise, lipoproteins and coronary artery disease. *Circulation* 79:1143-1145.

Kuipers, H. 1991. Overtraining. *Geneeskunde en Sport* 24930:90-94.

Kuipers, H. 1992. *Wielrennen.* Haarlem, The Netherlands: De Vrieseborch.

Kuipers, H., and H. A. Keizer. 1988. Overtraining in elite athletes. *Sports Medicine* 6:79-92.

Kulberg, B. J., and J. W. M. van der Meer. 1988. Het zal wel een virus zijn. *Nederlands Tijdschrift van geneeskunde* 132:193-195.

Lampe, J. W., J. L. Slavin, and F. S. Apple. 1986. Poor iron status of women runners training for a marathon. *International Journal of Sports Medicine* 7:111-114.

Lamont, L. S. Lack of influence of the menstrual cycle on blood lactate. *Physician and Sportsmedicine* 14:159-163.

Leinders, G., and P. Leinders. 1989. Het gebruik van lactaat onderzoek in de sportmedische praktijk.

Levine, B. D., and J. Stray-Gundersen. 1997. "Living high—training low": Effect of moderate altitude acclimatization with low-altitude training on performance. *Journal of Applied Physiology* 83:102-103.

Liesen, H. von. 1985. Trainungssteuerung im Hochleistungssport: Einige Aspekte und Beispiele. *Deutsche Zeitschrift für Sportmedizin* 1.

Liesen, H., and W. Hollmann. 1981. *Ausdauersport und Stoffwechsel*. Schorndorf.

Mader, A. et al. 1978. Evaluation of lactic acid anaerobic energy contribution by determination of post-exercise lactic concentration of ear capillary blood in middle-distance runners and swimmers. *Exercise Physiology*, 4:187-200.

Maron, B., A. Pelliccia, and P. Spirito. 1995. Cardiac disease in young trained athletes. *Circulation* 91(5):1596-1601.

Maron, B. J., ed. 1992. *Cardiology clinics—the athlete's heart*. Philadelphia: Saunders.

Martin, et al. 1997. Blood testing for professional cyclists. *Sports Science News.*

Mattner, U. 1987. *Lactate in sportsmedicine*. Mannheim, Germany: Boehringer.

Mellerowicz, H. 1977. Training. Lochem: De Tijdstroom.

Morgan, D. W., R. J. Cruise, B. W. Girardin, et al. 1986 HDL-C concentrations in weight-trained, endurance-trained and sedentary females. *Physician and Sportsmedicine* 14:166-181.

Mosimann, R., J. Walder, and G. van Melle. 1985. Stenotic thickening of the external iliac artery: Illness of the competition cyclist? *Vascular Surgery* 19:258-263.

Nelissen, P. C. 1995. Voeding bij sport. *Sportmassage International* 36(10):21-29.

Neumann, H. et al. 1993. *Alles unter Kontrolle*. Ausdauertraining Aachen, Meyer und Meyer.

NEVO-tabel. 1993. *Voorlichtingsbureau voor de Voeding*. The Hague, The Netherlands.

Noakes, T. D. 1993. Fluid replacement during exercise. *Exercise and Sport Sciences Reviews* 21:297-330.

Nonella, L. 1986. *Feldtest zur Ermittlung der anaeroben Schwelle*. Der Läufer.

Olbrecht, J. 1985. Relationship between swimming velocity and lactic concentration during continuous and intermittent training exercises. *International Journal of Sports Medicine* 6:74-77.

Olbrecht, J., et al 1984. De praktische betekenis van lactaatonderzoekingen voor trainingsplanning en trainingsuitvoering. Lezing te Diepenhout op 10 November 1984. Publicatie in Sportmedische Tijdingen. Tijdschrift van de Vlaamse vereniging van specialisten in de sportgeneeskunde (VVSS).

Olbrecht, J., et al. Vergleichende Untersuchungen des Laktatgeschwindigkeitsverhaltens im Zweistreckentest uber 400m Krawlschwimmen zum 30- und 60- minutigen maximalen und 30- minutigen submaximalen Schwimmen. *Deutsche Zeitschrift für Sportmedicin* 1:3-8.

Paffenbarger, R. S. Jr., R. T. Hyde, A. L. Wing, and C. C. Hsieh. 1986. Physical activity, all-cause mortality, and longevity of college alumni. *New England Journal of Medicine* 314:605-613.

Paffenbarger, R. S. Jr., R. T. Hyde, A. L. Wing, and C. H. Steinmetz. 1984. A natural history of athleticism and cardiovascular health. *Journal of the American Medical Association* 252:491-495.

Paffenbarger, R. S. Jr., A. L. Wing, and R. T. Hyde. 1978. Physical activity as an index of heart attack risk in college alumni. *American Journal of Epidemiology* 108:161-175.

Parisotto, R., C. J. Gore, K. R. Emslie, M. J. Ashenden, C. Brugnara, C. Howe, D. T. Martin, G. J. Trout, and A. G. Hahn. 2000. A novel method utilizing markers of altered erythropoiesis for the detection of recombinant human erythropoietine abuse in athletes. *Haematologica* 85:564-572.

Peters, H. P. F., W. F. van Schelven, P. A. Verstappen, R. W. de Boer, E. Bol, W. B. M. Erich, C. R. van der Togt, and W. R. de En Vries. 1995. Het sporthart in de jaren negentig. Koolhydraatrijke voeding; invloed op het optreden van maag- en darmklachten en het prestatievermogen tijdens langdurige inspanning. *Geneeskunde en Sport* 28(1):8-17.

Pluim, B. 1993. Het sporthart in de jaren negentig. *Geneeskunde en Sport* 26(4):137-144.